DISTANCE LEARNING
for Profesionals in
HEARING HEALTH SCIENCES

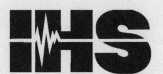

International Hearing Society
16880 Middlebelt Road, Suite 4
Livonia, Michigan 48154

Table of Contents

Foreword

The International Institute for Hearing Instruments Studies fundamental responsibility is to provide educational support and opportunities to the members of the International Hearing Society (formerly the National Hearing Aid Society) and those individuals who wish to enter or further their knowledge in the field of hearing instrument sciences. Toward this end, the Institute publishes a series of textbooks, sponsors educational courses, and supports continuing educational activities. Over the years one of the primary instruments for providing entry into the field of hearing instrument dispensing has been the Institute's Basic Course For Independent Study Of Hearing Aid Audiology.

The First Edition of the Basic Course was published in 1961, primarily through the efforts of two dedicated dispensers, Thornton Zanolli and Troy V. Grady. Both of these individuals were Certified Hearing Aid Audiologists as well as leaders and forward thinkers in the field of hearing health care. They perceived the need for an entry level vehicle to teach the fundamentals of hearing aid technology to those entering the field. These two individuals working with the Education Committee of the Society of Hearing Aid Audiologists (predecessor to the National Heating Aid Society) designed and published the first Basic Course.

The Basic Course has gone through four revisions during its history. The first revision was in 1967 with additional revisions in 1979 and 1986. Each time the course was revised to update and expand the information provided, to reflect advancements in technology and our understanding of the field of hearing sciences.

The Basic Course was designed as a self-paced independent study program. The course is considered only the first step in a continuous learning process, which must be pursued throughout the individual's career in the field of hearing health care. With these factors in mind the Institute reviewed the current Fourth Edition of the Basic Course and felt it was no longer meeting the needs of individuals wishing entry into our field. A new vehicle was needed which would cover the latest advances in the field of technology and science of modern hearing instrument dispensing. Towards this end the Institute redefined what knowledge a person entering our field should know to have a good foundation upon which to build a continuous learning process.

It is with pride and reverence that the International Institute for Hearing Instruments Studies now retires the Basic Course. The work started by Thornton Zanolli and Troy Grady does not stop with the retirement of the Basic Course. These individuals, and those that followed, developed not a textbook – but a vehicle of learning for those entering our field. This vehicle of learning is being continued with the Institute's new **Distance Learning for Professionals in Hearing Health Sciences.** The Training Manual along with the supporting textbooks published by the Institute provide a strong foundation upon which people entering our field can build their careers.

We acknowledge with gratitude the assistance of the many people involved in developing this new Training Manual to replace the Basic Course. Our special thanks go to C. Elaine Kramar, BC-HIS for taking on the task of providing material for this new manual. I also wish to thank the members of the Institute's Board of Directors, John (Jack) Young, Jr., Ernest Zelnick, Ph.D., John Roberts, Linda Donaldson, M.A., Larry Farris, and Jay McSpaden, Ph.D. To Phyllis V. Wilson, Administrative Director of the Institute, goes a very special thanks for her diligence in seeing this project was completed on time. I also wish to thank those pioneers who's foresight lead the way and set our current and future direction.

Jay H. Thurman, BC-HIS

First Edition 1993
Revised Edition 2000
Second Revision Edition 2002
Fourth Edition 2005
Fifth Edition 2008

INTERNATIONAL INSTITUTE FOR HEARING INSTRUMENTS STUDIES

DISTANCE LEARNING for PROFESSIONALS in HEARING HEALTH SCIENCES

*The **PATIENT** is the basic ingredient.*
Our knowledge, tests, measurements and hearing instrument
selection can be excellent in theory, but unless they satisfy the needs,
wants and desires of the patient to communicate better and improve
the quality of life, we have achieved nothing.

Introduction

This manual attempts to introduce and explain new information in an orderly fashion so it is easy to understand. Some of the reading material is not as basic. Loaded information creates an 'overwhelming' condition. This can become easier with a few working definitions. For instance, when you turn up the **volume** on the radio, it becomes **louder.**

The following terms relate to volume or loudness:

Amplitude	Intensity	Loudness
Sensation Level (SL)	Decibel (dB)	Volume

Volume is measured in **decibels (dB),** although the above terms apply as well. A decibel is a ratio. There are several different kinds of decibels for you to learn. For now, consider 140 dB to be extremely loud and 0 dB so quiet that you may not hear it.

Another example: A man's voice sounds deeper or lower in **frequency** than a woman's voice, even though they are speaking at the same volume. Frequency differences are grouped in **octaves,** just like music. Many other words are used in the same context:

Cycles per second (cps)	Octaves	Hertz (Hz)
Pitch	KiloHertz (KHz)	Tone

Frequency differences are measured in **cycles per second** or Hertz and arranged numerically in octaves. An **octave** is the interval between two frequencies when the higher is double the lower frequency.

For example, from 125 Hz to 250 Hz is one octave; from 2000 Hz to 4000 Hz is one octave. 500 Hz to 2000 Hz is two octaves. KHz is a Hz abbreviation - 5000 Hz is 5 KHz; 500 Hz is .5 KHz. Just move the decimal point three places to the left.

You will learn the exact definitions and differences between terms as we progress through the lessons.

A quiz follows each lesson, so the knowledge becomes a useful tool in your practice.

Completion of this course is just the beginning of one of the most rewarding occupations on the planet. Its ingredients are wonderful people of all ages, educational opportunities at a time when technology is on the brink of incredible advances for the benefit of mankind, an occupation where every day is different, rewarding, and challenging - where being there can and does make a difference to you and to those you touch.

Abbreviations

Abbreviations are also very common in the literature. Many are used on a daily basis.
Keep this list handy when you are reading. Most of them will easily become part of your vocabulary.
Add new terms as you encounter them.

AC	Air Conduction		Ln	Equivalent Input Noise Level
AGC	Automatic Gain Control		LL	Loudness Level
ALD	Assistive Listening Device		MCT	Minimum Contact Technology
ANSI	American National Standards Institute		MCL	Most Comfortable Loudness
ASP	Automatic Signal Processer		MSP	Multiple Signal Processer
AVC	Automatic Volume Control		n	Number (of subjects involved in a test)
BC	Bone Conduction		NAEL	National Assoc. of Earmold Laboratories
BTE	Behind-the-ear hearing instrument		NR	No Response
CFA	Continuous Flow Adapter (earmold)		OD	Outside Diameter (usually tubing)
CL	Comfortable Level		PB	Phonetically Balanced
CNS	Central Nervous System		PTA	Pure Tone Average
CNT	Can Not Test		PTS	Permanent Threshold Shift
CPS	Cycles Per Second		REAR	Real ear aided response
CROS	Contralateral Routing of Signals		REIG	Real ear insertion gain
dB	Decibel		REIR	Real ear insertion response
dBA	Decibels on A Scale of a sound level meter		REOR	Real ear occluded response
DNR	Did Not Respond		REUR	Real ear unaided response
DNT	Did Not Test		RMS	Root mean square (a composite tone)
DR	Dynamic Range		RTG	Reference Test Gain
DS	Discrimination Score		RTP	Reference Test Position
ENT	Ear, Nose and Throat Specialist		SAT	Speech Awareness Threshold
EM	Effective Masking		SAV	Select-a-vent
FF	Free Field		SDS	Speech Discrimination Score
FOG	Full on Gain		SDT	Speech Detection Threshold
HAE	Hearing Aid Evaluation		SF	Sound Field
HD	Harmonic Distortion		SIL	Speech Interference Level
HFA	High Frequency Average		SISI	Short Increment Sensitivity Index
HL	Hearing Level		SL	Sensation Level
HTL	Hearing Threshold Level		SLM	Sound Level Meter
	(re: Audiometric Zero)		S/N	Signal to Noise
Hz	Hertz		SPL	Sound Pressure Level
IA	Interaural Attenuation		SRT	Speech Reception Threshold
ID	Inside Diameter (usually tubing)		SSPL	Saturation Sound Pressure Level
IE	In-the-ear hearing instrument		TD	Threshold of Discomfort
IL	Intensity Level		THD	Total Harmonic Distortion
IM	Intermodulation Distortion		TL	Tolerance Level
IHS	International Hearing Society		TM	Tympanic Membrane
JND	Just Noticeable Difference		TMJ	Temporomandibular Joint
KEMAR	Knowles Electronic Manikin for		TTS	Temporary Threshold Shift
	Acoustical Research		UCL	Uncomfortable Loudness
KHz	Kilohertz		VU	VU Meter on Audiometer

INTERNATIONAL INSTITUTE FOR HEARING INSTRUMENTS STUDIES

DISTANCE LEARNING for Professionals in HEARING HEALTH SCIENCES

IIHIS

Unit I - The Human Ear

CONTENTS

This unit will examine the anatomy, physiology, disorders, diseases and acoustic properties of the ear.

Anatomy reviews the structures of the ear. Physiology describes how these parts work together to transmit and convert sound. Diseases and disorders affect either the hearing mechanism directly, or the entire body, including hearing. Acoustics is the science of sound as it relates to hearing.

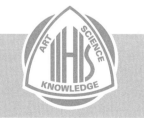

Published by
International Institute for Hearing Instruments Studies
Educational Division of International Hearing Society

The human ear has two important functions. The first, and best known, is hearing. This involves the Auditory System which divides into three parts: The External Ear, The Middle Ear and the Inner Ear. The second function concerns balance and equilibrium. The Vestibular System influences our eye movement and body positioning as we change our movements in space. Except for the outer ear, the structures of the ear are within the temporal bone of the skull.

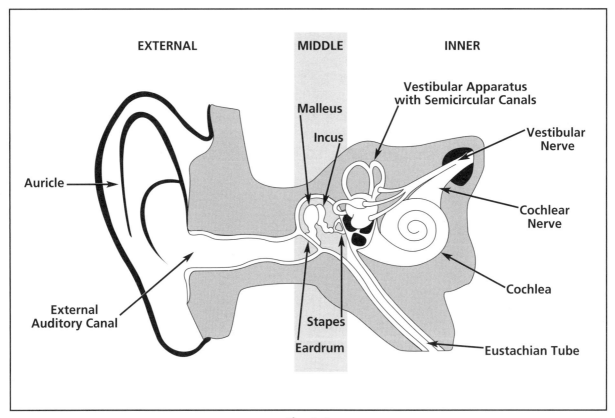

Fig. 1-1
The Human Ear

When most people think about the human ear, they visualize the fleshy part that protrudes from the side of a person's head.

This part, the **auricle** or **pinna,** is only one part of the ear. Most of the ear's delicate, complicated mechanism lies hidden in deep cavities in the skull. The outer ear is the least important part of the hearing mechanism, but it is the critically important part in the proper fitting of a hearing instrument. Almost all fittings require the hearing instrument to be on or in the ear.

The curves and convolutions of the pinna collect and funnel acoustic energy (sound) into the ear canal

Normally, both ears (**pinnae**) work together to locate the original sound source, the direction of the sound, and separate one sound from another.

The pinna consists of **cartilage,** covered with skin. There is a vast difference in the cartilage texture from person to person. The cartilage supporting the pinna varies from extremely stiff and rigid on one person to soft and malleable on another.

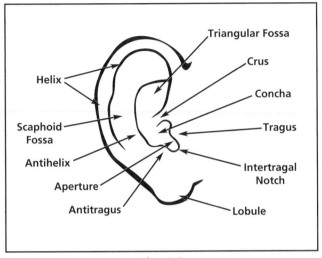

Fig. 1-2
Auricle

The blood vessels in the pinna are not plentiful and do not have much of a protective layer of fat. It is easy for the pinna to become frostbitten in extremely cold weather.

The outer edge or fold of the auricle is the **helix.** The inner raised area or rim is the **antihelix.** The **crus** of the helix overlaps the antihelix at the upper front edge. Near the top of the auricle, between the helix and antihelix, is the **triangular fossa.** The bulk of the rear outer curved area is the **scaphoid fossa.** The lower tip of the ear is the **lobule** or **ear lobe.** The **tragus** is the outward projection or bump on the front of the ear that is suspended over the ear canal. The bump or projection on the back part of the inner rim is the **antitragus.** Between the tragus and antitragus is the **intertragal notch,** which forms the bottom of the inner rim. The **concha** is the small hollow or bowl leading directly into the ear canal. The **aperture** is the entrance to the canal. The canal, itself, is the **external auditory meatus.** It extends from the concha inward to the **eardrum** or **tympanic membrane.**

THE EAR CANAL

The **external auditory meatus** or **ear canal** is not usually straight. It curves like a figure 'S', laying on its side. In adults, it rises slightly upward, then slightly forward and downward toward the eardrum.

The outer portion of the canal contains tiny hairs (**cilia**), wax producing **ceruminous glands** and **sebaceous** (oil) **glands.** Here, a thick skin covers **cartilage,** while the inner portion has a thinner skin that lines **temporal bone.**

The canal is normally a self-cleaning mechanism. The skin grows outward from the eardrum to the outer canal. The fine hairs gently and constantly move dry particles of **cerumen** (wax), and sloughed skin, into the concha bowl.

The **size** of a normal ear canal varies in length, width and direction. In adults, the length varies from about 2.3 cm (1 inch), to 2.9 cm (1 3/8 inches). It is about 0.7 cm (almost 1/4 inch) in diameter, the diameter of an ordinary lead pencil. Half-way between the external opening and the eardrum, the canal becomes quite narrow as it enters the temporal bone. This narrow area is the **isthmus.** Beyond the isthmus, the canal again opens to its original diameter. The isthmus is just past the **second bend** when making ear impressions.

The ear canal is warm and moist, maintaining a fairly constant temperature and humidity. Many hospitals use a specula in the ear canal, similar to an otoscope, to determine body temperature in seconds.

EAR CANAL RESONANCE

Ear canal resonance is an important function of the ear canal. The canal ends at the eardrum, forming a tube, closed at one end. Any open or closed tube has a natural resonant frequency. The ear canal is no exception.

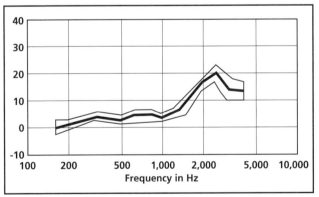

Fig. 1-3
Natural Ear Canal Resonance

Ear canals vary in both length and diameter. Sounds entering the ear are naturally enhanced by the resonance of the canal. Resonance varies slightly from person to person because of the individual sizes and shapes.

Most ear canals resonate between 2000 to 3000 Hz. The average resonant frequency is about 2700 Hz. This average is a combination of the pinna, which resonates between 2000 - 5000 Hz.

A branch of the **Vagus Nerve (X Cranial)** lies along the bottom of the canal, between the outer opening and the isthmus. Often this nerve is touched, using Q-Tips, making ear impressions, or using an earmold or hearing instrument, causing an automatic cough, - Arnold's Reflex. Approximately one person in seven reacts, but not necessarily on both ears.

THE EARDRUM

The eardrum, called the **tympanic membrane** or **tympanum** or **drumhead**, is the dividing line between the outer and middle ear.

It is **oval** in shape, slightly convex, like a cone with the hollow part of the cone facing outward, and at a 30 degree angle to the bottom of the canal. Normal color is translucent, pearly white to pinkish grey. You can usually see through it.

The **size** of the eardrum is about 9mm (l/4 inch) high, and 8 mm (3/8 inch) wide, the size of the hole made by a large paper punch. The drum membrane is as thin as tissue paper and extremely strong. It has three layers. The first is the **skin** of the ear canal which also lines the eardrum's outer surface. Next, is a tough **fibrous layer.** The outermost fibers are like the spokes of a wheel. The inner fibers are concentric, radiating in ever expanding circles. Together, they form an extremely strong grid, giving the membrane durability under pressure, like water, air, and infection, without ripping or tearing most of the time. And, third is the inner layer called the **mucous membrane**, which lines the middle ear cavity.

In children, the eardrum is thin and elastic, becoming thicker and more rigid in adults. The **annulus** or **annular ring** holds the eardrum in place, forming a watertight and airtight seal between the external and middle ear.

Vibrations of sound, **acoustic energy**, enhanced by pinna and ear canal resonances, cause the eardrum to move back and forth in response to these vibrations. The eardrum is attached to the malleus in the middle ear.

In normal ears, the **malleus** is suspended from the top of the eardrum to a point about 2/3 of the way down the drum. At the point where the tip of the malleus ends, **the umbo,** the eardrum is pulled in toward the middle ear, forming the innermost tip of the cone.

Light from an otoscope reflects from the umbo to the bottom of the drum. This reflected light is the **cone of light,** and is present in varying degrees on most normal drums.

The tissue on the lower four-fifths of the drum is tight, and is the **pars tensa**. The upper fifth, loose or more flaccid because it lacks most of the fibrous layer, is the **pars flaccida**.

QUADRANTS OF THE EARDRUM

The eardrum is divided into four sections or quadrants to help us to better describe the location of anatomical parts or areas of concern.

Consider the eardrum to be a circle on the side of the head. The vertical axis follows the malleus manubrium, starting in the one o'clock position, giving you a back (posterior) and a front (anterior) view. The horizontal axis starts at the four o'clock position. The top half of the circle becomes superior, and the bottom, inferior.

This division now overlaps itself. For instance, a hole in the posterior-superior quadrant narrows down where to find the hole.

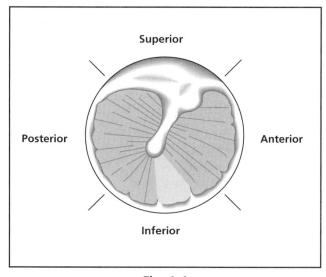

Fig. 1-4
Right Drum

HOW TO PRONOUNCE THE
TECHNICAL TERMS USED IN THIS LESSON

Annulus	An' u-lus	Mastoid	mass-toyd'
Aperture	Ap'-er-cher	Meatus	me-a'tus
Antihelix	an"tǐ-he'-liks	Mucous	mu'-kus
Antitragus	an" tǐ-tra'-gus	Pars Flaccida	pars flak'-ši dah
Auricle	aw' rě-kl	Pars Tensa	pars ten'-suh
Cerumen	sě-roo' men	Petrous	pet'-rus
Ceruminous	sě-roo'-mi-nus	Pinna	pin'-nah
Concha	kong-kah	Scaphoid	skaf' oyd
Crus	krus	Squamous	skwa' mus
Fossa	fah-sah	Temporal	temp' uh-rehl
Helix	he'-licks	Tragus	tra'-gus
Intertragal	in-ter-tray'-gull	Tympanic	tim-pan'-ik
Isthmus	is'-mas	Tympanum	tim' pah-num
Malleus	mal'e-us	Umbo	um' bo
Manubrium	ma-noo'-bree-um	Vagus	vay' gus

DISORDERS OF THE OUTER EAR

LESSON 2

*The Hearing Instrument Specialist who provides the hearing instrument **should not, in any way, attempt to diagnose, or state the cause of a hearing inpairment, or attempt any treatment or medical advice**. Diagnosis, and the medical or surgical treatment of hearing loss, is the special task of the physician.*

You require a basic knowledge of hearing disorders for four reasons:

1. To add to your knowledge of the workings of the hearing mechanism;
2. To help you to understand the medical problems of your client;
3. To enable you to know when to refer your client to a physician;
4. To help you to better select amplification appropriate to the specific loss of your client.

TYPES of HEARING LOSS

1. A **conductive hearing loss** involves the breakdown or obstruction of some part of the **external** or **middle ear.** The physical vibrations of sound are no longer transmitted or conducted through air, bone or tissue because of the obstruction. Most problems are medically correctable.
2. A **sensorineural hearing loss** results in damage occurring in the **inner ear**.
3. A **mixed hearing loss** is a combination of more than one type of loss, usually conductive and sensorineural.
4. A **central hearing loss** is the inability of the **brain** to process, recognize or understand sounds or speech accurately.
5. A **non-organic hearing loss**, often called 'functional loss', is a result of some sort of **psychological** cause. There is nothing physically wrong with a person's hearing mechanism.

Although you cannot diagnose, or state the cause of a hearing loss, you must be able to recognize the types of loss. Hearing instrument requirements are vastly different according to the loss. Amplification is not indicated for the individual with non-organic hearing loss. Also, often it is not successful for clients with central hearing loss.

The following conditions indicate conductive disorders. All conductive disorders **require referral to a physician:**

Malformations of the ear, include **atresia** (closure) of the external auditory canal and malformed or missing auricle, 'cauliflower ear.' These malformations may cause hearing loss.

Impacted cerumen is a common cause of conductive loss. Normally, the cerumen moves outward to the entrance of the external ear canal. Sometimes, cerumen accumulates in the canal, forming a plug, which partly or completely blocks the canal. The plug is a brown, yellow, or reddish mass if it is wet, or a black mass if it is hard and dry, (common in the older population). If the blockage is partial, there is little or no hearing loss. If the blockage is complete, or impacted, loss always occurs. Do not test or fit a hearing instrument until the physician removes the ceruminous plug.

Wax coating the eardrum can restrict its movement, causing some hearing loss, before removal by a physician.

Eczema or dermatitis makes the external ear (auricle) itchy and painful. The skin of the external auditory canal becomes red and swollen. This condition will not cause a hearing loss unless the swelling blocks the canal. Refer to a physician. Testing can be done, if the swelling does not block the canal.

Otitis externa is an inflammation of the walls of the external auditory canal which will not cause a hearing loss unless the swelling blocks the canal.

Polyps are masses of tissue that grow outward from a surface. Any polyp, lump or bony growth is a cause for referral.

Prolapsed canal, associated with the aging process, is a breakdown or sag of tissue around the canal. It causes the walls of the canal to collapse. A flap of tissue can partially or completely block the external canal. The canal will open up by lifting the pinna upward and backward.

Perforations or ruptures are holes in the eardrum. They are caused by infection, a foreign object, a bone fracture, a nearby explosion, or a blow on the ear with the palm of the hand. Small perforations cause a 10 to 15 dB loss in hearing sensitivity. Small holes often heal in a few weeks. Larger perforations require a surgical technique, **tympanoplasty or myringoplasty,** to 'patch' the hole.

Fluid drainage of any kind, whether odorous or clear, requires referral.

Monomeric spots look like a hole, but they reflect light from an otoscope, like a mirror. These spots are holes that have healed and are only one layer thick. They are called 'mirror membranes' as well.

A tumor or **cholesteatoma,** occurring in the middle ear, sometimes perforates the upper portion of the eardrum, invading the external auditory canal. There is a constant odorous discharge. A person with these symptoms requires immediate referral to a physician.

An **enlarged canal** is a result of ear surgery. Often these clients have no eardrum or ossicular chain in the middle ear. The skin of the ear canal can be very sensitive. If the eardrum is missing, approval of a physician is required before fitting a hearing instrument.

Often, when a perforation heals or the ear has had +recurring infections, **the drum itself can become scarred.** This restricts its movement and can create a small conductive loss.

Tympanosclerosis is white, chalky calcium deposits, caused by a degeneration of the tissue on the eardrum.

Foreign objects in the ear canal can range from cotton wads, erasers, insects, sprouting wheat and assorted unpredictable items.

HOW TO PRONOUNCE THE TECHNICAL TERMS USED IN THIS LESSON

Atresia	ah-tre' ze-ah
Cholesteatoma	ko" le-ste" ah-to' mah
Dermatitis	der-mah-tight'-us
Eczema	eg-zee'-mah
Monomeric	mahn'-oh-mer'-ic
Otitis externa	o-ti' tis x-ter'-nah
Polyp	paw'-lip
Sensorineural	sen" so-re-nu' ral
Tympanosclerosis	tim"pah'-no-skleĕ-ro'sis

THE MIDDLE EAR OR TYMPANIC CAVITY

LESSON 3

The middle ear is a mucous membrane lined, air-filled space, hollowed out of the temporal bone. It contains three tiny bones with their ligaments, two muscles, the opening of the Eustachian tube, the oval window and the round window. The attic of the middle ear, or **epitympanic cavity,** has an opening which allows air into the mastoid air cells of the temporal bone. Branches of several nerves travel though the middle ear in protected passageways or tunnels in the bone.

The boundaries of the middle ear are the tympanic membrane and the oval window. Remember, the third layer of the tympanic membrane is mucous membrane, which lines all of the middle ear. Mucous membrane is a thin layer of tissue containing fluid secreting cells.

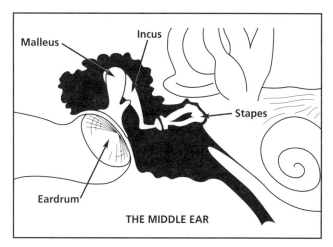

Fig. 3-1
The Middle Ear

The **ossicles** are the smallest bones in the human body. You probably know them by their English names - the hammer, anvil and stirrup. Their Latin names, in the same order, are **malleus, incus and stapes.**

These bones are suspended by ligaments, and loosely connected to each other to form a linkage known as the **ossicular chain.** The manubrium (handle) of the malleus is attached to the eardrum. The top of the malleus articulates with the top of the incus; the bottom of the incus meets the head of the stapes to form the **incudostapedial junction.** The footplate of the stapes is held in the oval window by the **annular ligament.**

This linkage permits the transmission of acoustic energy from the eardrum to the oval window using a lever principle - **mechanical energy.**

The middle ear is a **transducer.** A transducer changes energy from one form to another. The middle ear transduces **acoustic energy** from the eardrum to **mechanical energy** in the ossicular chain. The stapes footplate transduces mechanical energy from the ossicular chain to **hydraulic energy** in the inner ear.

The middle ear is also a **transformer** because it causes an increase in sound pressure to occur. The eardrum is roughly 17 times larger than the oval window. The ossicular chain, acting as a lever, increases the sound pressure delivered to the oval window by approximately 1.3 times. The **transfer function** or areal ratio of the middle ear is about **22:1,** (17 x 1.3 = 22), an increase of 27 dB.

The tensor tympani and stapedius muscles are the smallest in the human body. The **tensor tympani** attaches to the handle of the malleus. The smaller **stapedius** attaches to the neck of the stapes. The other end of each muscle joins to a wall of the middle ear cavity.

These muscles have two purposes:

(1) They keep the bone linkage taut so that it can respond appropriately to vibrations, and

(2) They prevent extreme motions of the linkage which might result in damage from very loud sounds. If damage does occur, **ossicular discontinuity** results. The ossicles no longer articulate properly, and the lever action is reduced or eliminated.

When a loud sound from the outer ear is received by the middle ear, the tensor tympani and stapedius muscles contract, causing the ossicular chain to stiffen or move out of alignment with each other. This movement prevents sound from being amplified in the same relationship, and, in effect, puts a damper on the system. The involuntary response or contraction of the stapes is **acoustic reflex**. When the stapedius contracts in one ear, it also contracts in the other, even if the opposite ear did not hear the loud sound. Stapedial acoustic reflex can be measured with an impedance bridge.

The **oval window** is an opening in the bone between the air-filled middle ear and the fluid filled inner ear. It is covered by a thin membrane. The footplate of the stapes is set in the oval window, over the membrane, and both are sealed in the window by an annular ligament. Sound is transmitted from the ossicular chain to the inner ear through this window.

The **round window** is a membrane covered opening in the bone, separating the middle and inner ear. Although the membrane is in the middle ear, its function is part of the inner ear.

The oval and round window are separated by a bony prominence, the **promontory.** This bulge is the wall of the cochlea in the inner ear.

The **Eustachian tube,** also called the auditory tube, runs from the lower part of the middle ear cavity to the upper part of the throat. This area, behind the nose, is the **nasopharynx.** The nasopharynx provides a direct connection for outside air to enter the middle ear through the Eustachian tube.

If the Eustachian tube cannot function properly, or at all, then the middle ear remains in a negative pressure, or a partial vacuum. The tympanic membrane retracts. The ossicular chain no longer functions. Negative pressure draws fluid from the mucous membrane lining into the middle ear cavity. Conductive hearing loss results.

Children have a rather straight, short, horizontal, relatively open, Eustachian tube. Germs can readily pass from the nasopharynx to the middle ear through this open tube, causing infection. The tube is horizontal, so fluid drainage from the middle ear is not ideal.

Adults have a longer, arched, downward slanting Eustachian tube. It is about 3.7 cm (1 1/2 inches) long, normally closed, preventing infection and enhancing fluid drainage. In adults, the tube is **patent,** meaning it opens during such actions as a cough, sneeze or swallow. These actions permit air to travel from the outside to the middle ear, or from the middle ear to the outside, depending on which is necessary to equalize the air pressure on the outside of the eardrum.

HOW TO PRONOUNCE THE
TECHNICAL TERMS USED IN THIS LESSON

Eustachian	u-sta' shun
Incudostapedial	ink" u-do-sta-pe' de-al
Incus	ink' us
Nasopharynx	na" zo-far' inks
Ossicle	os-si'-kul
Ossicular	os-si'-ku-ler
Patent	pa' tent
Stapedius	stah-pe'-de-us
Stapes	sta' pēz
Tensor Tympani	ten' sor tim-pah' ne

A **conductive** hearing loss involves the breakdown or obstruction of some part of the external or middle ear which transmits or conducts the physical vibrations of sound through air, bone or tissue. The following are conductive disorders. **These require referral to a physician**.

Otitis media is the presence of fluid in the middle ear. This fluid may be a thin, watery, sterile fluid, or mucous or pus (purulent). Otitis media is much more common in children than in adults.

Suppurative otitis media is an infection of the middle ear, usually caused by bacteria from a cold or other respiratory infection. Germs enter the middle ear through the Eustachian tube. The Eustachian tube becomes blocked, trapping fluid in the middle ear cavity. The disease may be **acute** (severe, but of short duration) or **chronic** (recurring or lasting a long time). In the acute stage, pus collects in the middle ear cavity and causes hearing loss. The pressure of the pus causes pain. The eardrum appears bright red instead of its normal pinkish-gray color.

Acute suppurative otitis media is treated with antibiotics, or by a **myringotomy,** an incision in the eardrum to allow drainage. Often, a tube is temporarily placed in this incision. This tube ventilates the middle ear cavity, and will fall out after a few months, leaving a small perforation. Normally, this perforation heals itself. Without treatment, the pressure of the pus ruptures the eardrum, causing a perforation, and allows the pus to drain into the ear canal. When this occurs, the pain is relieved. The perforation can usually heal itself.

When treated by antibiotics alone, sometimes the symptoms of earache, fever, and drainage seem to be completely controlled by the antibiotic. The patient appears to make a complete recovery until hearing loss is noticed. Fluid remains trapped in the middle ear, but is now sterile because of the antibiotics. The Eustachian tube remains blocked, causing **serous otitis media or middle ear effusion.** This important cause of acquired hearing loss is progressive, and very often overlooked.

When infection occurs repeatedly, it is **chronic suppurative otitis media**, or 'running ear.' The perforation in the pars tensa portion of the eardrum will not heal. Infection erodes some parts of the ossicular chain; scar tissue also causes hearing loss, further impeding the action of the ossicular chain. This loss is usually permanent. With the passage of time, the perforation becomes larger. This type of perforation rarely produces a cholesteatoma.

Chronic suppurative otitis media is more difficult to treat. If the perforation is not too large, a **tympanoplasty** repairs the ossicular chain, or replaces diseased bones with a prosthesis, and grafts skin over the eardrum. This stops the progression of the hearing loss, and eliminates the constant discharge.

If the mastoid air cells have also become infected, a **mastoidectomy** is performed, removing diseased mastoid cells, prior to a tympanoplasty.

Sometimes, the diseased area requires removal of the ossicular chain and mastoid air cells, a **radical mastoidectomy**. This operation creates a permanent conductive hearing loss, but stops further deterioration and can be life-saving.

Non-suppurative otitis media is also called **areo-otitis media, serous otitis media, middle ear effusion, mucoid otitis media, or 'glue ear'.** It is similar to suppurative otitis media, except the fluid occurring in the middle ear, or the Eustachian tube, contains no bacteria because of antibiotic treatment. In other words, it is not pus; it is serum or mucus. It sounds safer, but it isn't, because it can go undetected for a long time.

Aero-otitis media, or barotrauma, occurs when the Eustachian tube does not open properly, for example, after an airplane flight, or while skin diving. Serous fluid (serum) collects in the middle ear. The drum appears normal, but with a bluish or yellowish light reflex. Often, a fluid line or bubbles show behind the drum.

Mucoid otitis media, middle ear effusion, or 'glue ear.' A cold, allergy, or respiratory infection, blocks the Eustachian tube and traps fluid in the middle ear. Antibiotic treatment destroys the bacteria, but the fluid remains trapped because of the plugged Eustachian tube. This fluid is mucous, a thick, gummy substance, produced by the mucous membranes. No inflammation occurs. The drum will appear normal, or opaque. Closer inspection shows a yellowish light reflex present, some fullness and often a fluid level or bubbles.

Treatment is usually a myringotomy, or inflation of the Eustachian tube to remove the fluid. If left untreated, this fluid can change the tissues of the mucous membrane lining, form scar tissue, and cause further hearing loss.

The negative pressure of the middle ear creates a partial vacuum and sucks in the eardrum until it drapes tightly over the ossicular chain. The eardrum tends to form pockets in the pars flaccida. These pockets produce a cholesteatoma and perforation of the eardrum. A person with any form of otitis media should not be fitted with a hearing instrument without referral to a physician.

Otosclerosis is a disease which causes spongy changes in the bony capsule surrounding the inner ear. Sometimes these changes will harden (that is, become sclerotic). Gradually, the footplate of the stapes becomes fixed, so the stapes loses its mobility. This causes a hearing loss of 60 to 65 dB, often accompanied by tinnitus. Otosclerosis occurs more often in women than in men and more often in caucasians than in other races. The disease is inherited, so otosclerosis may 'run in families.' Pregnancy often triggers the onset of otosclerosis.

Three surgical techniques have been used to treat cases of otosclerosis; fenestration (not used today), stapes mobilization and stapedectomy.

Ossicular discontinuity can occur in the presence of loud sound, slaps to the head, accidents, etc. The bones in the ossicular chain no longer fit together properly, altering the leverage capabilities of the middle ear.

Ossicular fixation can occur when ossification (the conversion of tissue to a bony substance) involves the ligaments of the ossicular chain. When this involves the eardrum, it is **tympanosclerosis.** This often occurs in people with osteoarthritis.

In Stapes Mobilization, the stapes footplate is directly manipulated, to free it from the new growth, and allow normal movement. A successful manipulation of the stapes eliminates the conductive component in the hearing loss. A decided disadvantage to this procedure is that often the otosclerosis again fixes the footplate, restricting movement.

In Stapedectomy a tiny plastic or steel strut (or piece of wire attached to gelfoam or fatty tissue) replaces the completely removed stapes. At present, this is the operation of choice by most ear surgeons. Successful surgery eliminates the conductive component in the hearing loss. The strut is attached to the bottom of the incus. Over time, it can cause the tip of the incus to break off. It is sometimes possible to have the strut moved higher up the incus. This creates a small hearing loss, compared to the first operation, but much better hearing than when the ossicular chain is no longer connected to the strut.

During a stapedectomy, the stapedius muscle, attached to the stapes, is severed, and is not re-attached. No 'damper' is on the system for protection in loud noise. Take care, when fitting a hearing instrument, to insure this protection.

In Fenestration the eardrum and most of the ossicles were removed and a tiny window (a fenestra), about the size of a grain of rice, was made through the bony wall into the horizontal semi-circular canal. A flap of skin was placed over this window. The new pathway for the sound was through the external auditory canal, directly through the middle ear to the fenestra, and through the fluid of the semi-circular canal to the fluid in the cochlea.

This operation is seldom used today since, with best results, about a 35 dB loss remains.

Cholesteatoma is a tumor occurring in the attic of the middle ear. It sometimes perforates the pars flaccida area of the eardrum, and invades the external auditory canal. A constant odorous discharge is present. Refer to a physician immediately. Removal of the tumor usually leaves some permanent conductive hearing loss.

Tinnitus or ringing in the ears is often present in conductive losses, usually a low frequency sound. Refer anyone with tinnitus to a physician.

Teeth missing, ill-fitting dentures, or clients who do not wear their teeth (edentulous) also create conductive losses. Often, the temporomandibular joint of the jaw is not in alignment, producing Eustachian tube problems and/or accompanying tinnitus.

Congenital problems (present at birth) can also create conductive losses. Cleft palate, or problems at birth are examples.

HOW TO PRONOUNCE THE
TECHNICAL TERMS USED IN THIS LESSON

Areo-otitis	Air'-oh o-ti' tis
Cholesteatoma	ko" le-ste" ah-to'mah
Fenestration	fen" es-tra'shun
Mastoidectomy	mas-toid-ek'-tah-me
Myringotomy	mir" in-got' o-me
Otosclerosis	o" to-skle-ro' sis
Stapedectomy	sta" pe-dek' to-me
Suppurative	su-per-a-tive
Tinnitus	ti-ni' tus
Tympanoplasty	tim" pah-no-plas' te

INNER EAR

The inner ear is not a removable structure that could stand alone, like the ossicular chain. It is a series of tunnels and cavities hollowed out of the petrous portion of the temporal bone. These tunnels and cavities are filled with two separate and continuous fluids from one portion to another. The outer fluid is always **perilymph fluid.** The inner fluid, which is separated by a membrane, is **endolymph fluid.** Although the inner ear is a continuous cavity, it is discussed as if it were three separate and distinct parts: semi-circular canals, vestibule and cochlea.

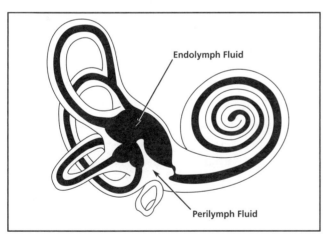

Fig. 5-1
Membranous Labyrinth

There are three semi-circular canals, Superior, Posterior and Lateral, oriented at 90 degrees to one another. The outer portion of these fluid filled ducts contains perilymph fluid, which protects the membranous endolymph fluid. These canals detect rotational movement in any direction for balance and equilibrium.

These canals serve no known hearing function. Balance problems and dizziness or vertigo can develop, along with hearing loss, as the fluids are continuous throughout the entire inner ear.

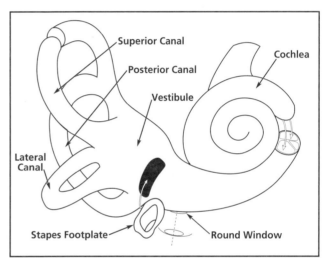

Fig. 5-2
Boney Labyrinth

The back part of each semicircular canal unites to form a common trunk, entering the vestibule. The front end of each semi-circular canal, closest to the middle ear, enlarges to form an ampulla (ampullae is plural), attached to the vestibule. There are three ampullae, superior, posterior and lateral, just like the canals.

VESTIBULE

The Vestibule is the tiny, irregularly-shaped space inside the oval window, behind the stapes footplate. The vestibule is just as its name implies, a meeting place for the semi-circular canals, the stapes footplate, and the cochlea.

The vestibule contains two membranous sacs from the semi-circular canals, the **utricle** at the top and the **saccule**, below. These contain endolymph fluid. Both ends of each semi-circular canal enter the utricle, the largest of the two connected sacs. The smaller saccule funnels into the cochlea, at the bottom of the vestibule. Perilymph fluid surrounds the saccule and utricle, and is the fluid behind the stapes footplate.

The ampullae, the utricle, and the saccule all contain sensory endings of the Vestibular Nerve, which becomes a branch of the Auditory Nerve.

COCHLEA

The cochlea coils around like a snail shell in 2 1/2 to 2 3/4 turns. The inside of this bony labyrinth sections off, but is not completely divided, into three parts by the (bony) **osseous spiral lamina** on the inside wall, and the **spiral ligament** on the outside wall.

These sections consist of three tapering tubes (scalae), in layers, one on top of the other. The two outer tubes, containing perilymph fluid, are the **scala vestibuli** on the top, and the **scala tympani** on the bottom. The middle, smaller, triangular shaped tube is the **scala media**. The **auditory nerve endings** are in the scala media, also called the **cochlear duct**, or **canal of the cochlea,** or **membranous labyrinth.** There is no fluid connection between the scala media and the scala vestibuli, or between the scala media and the scala tympani.

If we unwind the cochlea and part of the vestibule to straighten it out, as shown in the diagram, we get a better idea of the structures involved.

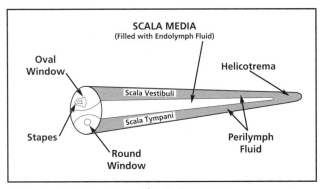

Fig. 5-3
Cochlea Fluids

The stapes footplate in the oval window vibrates the perilymph fluid in the upper scala, the **scala vestibuli.** The scala vestibuli and the **scala tympani** meet at the **helicotrema.** The round window, at the other end of the scala tympani, is directly below the stapes footplate. Between these two scalae, is the triangular **scala media**. Thin membranes completely encase and separate the scala media from the other scalae throughout the full length of the cochlea. The domed end of the scala media is the **cupola.**

The oval window, a small opening in the vestibular portion of the temporal bone, houses the stapes footplate. The mechanical action of the ossicular chain converts to fluid waves (hydraulic energy) in the perilymph fluid of the scala vestibuli.

The stapes footplate rocks in the oval window in response to the sound waves arriving from the eardrum. This creates a pressure wave through the fluid in the cochlea. The temporal bone is extremely hard, and will not 'give' at all, so this fluid must have somewhere to go when the stapes pushes the fluid inward.

The round window serves this function. The round window is a flexible membrane in the scala tympani. It allows the fluid movement from the scala vestibuli to distend the membrane outward. The membrane bulges into the middle ear, and inward again, as the stapes rocks back and forth.

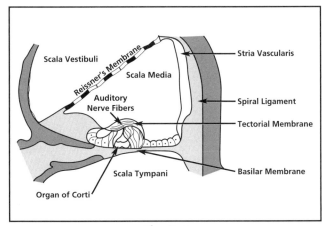

Fig. 5-4
Cross Section of Cochlea

The diagram of a cross-section of the cochlea allows you to see the smaller structures. **Reissner's membrane** separates the scala media from the scala vestibuli. The inside edge connects to the spiral lamina, and the outside to the spiral ligament.

Reissner's membrane is extremely thin - so thin, in fact, that it is almost as if it were not there at all. The scala media and the scala vestibuli are not connected. They even contain different types of fluid, endolymph and perilymph. Reissner's membrane is so thin that they behave as if they were a single fluid space.

The **basilar membrane** separates the scala media from the scala tympani. The basilar membrane is the base of the **Organ of Corti** in the scala media. It, too, is connected to the spiral lamina and the spiral ligament.

The basilar membrane is narrow and stiff at the oval window, becoming broader and more compliant as it progresses to the apical end (cupola).

The outer wall of the scala media is formed by the spiral ligament and the **stria vascularis.** This network of capillaries secretes endolymph fluid, and is the source of chemicals in the endolymph, necessary for hair cells to function.

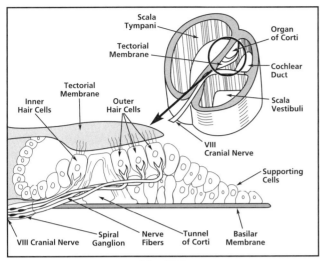

Fig. 5-5
Organ of Corti

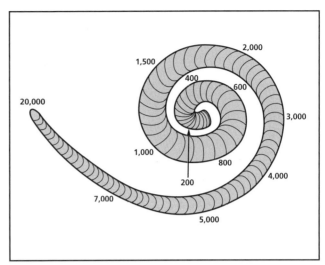

Fig. 5-6
Tonotopic Organization

The Organ of Corti consists of columns of **inner** and **outer rods** with **hair cells (cilia)** at the top of the rods. **Supporting cells** hold these rods and hair cells in place.

Although illustrations show only a few hairs in the cells, they are more like a hairbrush, with tufts of 40 hairs at the base of the cochlea, increasing to tufts of l00 at the apical end. There is one row of inner rods and three to five rows of outer rods depending upon the location in the cochlea.

The tectorial membrane, a gelatinous structure, attaches to the supporting cells at the inner side only, and is suspended over the hair cells. Tufts of the tops of the hair cells are embedded in the under side of the tectorial membrane.

Please note that all three membranes, basilar, Reissner's and tectorial, and the Organ of Corti run the full length of the scala media.

Any vibration through the surrounding fluid, or movement of the tectorial membrane, affects the hair cells. The fluid vibrations cause the tectorial membrane to undulate. A 'shearing action' takes place on the hair cells. The base of the hair cells contain nerve endings, converting this shearing action into **nerve impulses.** At this point, the nerve impulses become **electrical energy.**

The cochlea is often compared to a piano. The piano has only eighty-eight keys, while the cochlea, in effect, has thousands. The piano covers tones of a little more than seven octaves. The cochlea covers almost one octave lower than the piano and slightly more than two octaves higher.

The base of the cochlea, nearest to the oval window, responds to high frequencies. The part of the cochlea farthest away, at the apex, responds to low frequencies. Intermediate frequencies occur at intervals between the base and the apex.

HAIR CELLS

Hair cells are arranged in well defined rows, with about 3500 inner hair cells and 12,000 outer hair cells. The outer hair cells, believed to be 35 dB more sensitive than the inner hair cells, are damaged by loud sounds or ototoxic drugs.

The base of the hair cells contain **nerve endings,** which, when triggered or excited, become nerve impulses. **The Place Theory** says there are specific places in the cochlea, the pathways to the brain and the **temporal lobe,** itself, for specific frequencies. This is **tonotopic organization.** Each nerve fiber has a **tuning frequency,** and discharges more easily at that frequency than at any other.

The Volley Theory says that there are sequences of firing which allow for the transmission of neural energy from the inner ear to the brain at rates faster than any single nerve fibers could fire. By volleying, these fibers accomplish the desired rate in combination with each other. For example, several fibers firing in sequence permit higher frequencies to be achieved than single fibers could reach.

The Temporal Theory holds that at or below 1000 Hz, the place theory is correct. Above 1000 Hz, nerve fibers fire in **volleys.** They take turns firing. The combined total of these firings equals the specific frequency. The temporal theory also includes maximum amplitude of the wave on the Basilar Membrane, for resonance.

Most researchers agree that some combination of these three theories are used.

The loudness of a sound appears to relate to the **number** of nerve fibers that are stimulated, and to the **rate** of stimulation. The precise mechanism that the cochlea and the auditory nerve encode and transmit sound is not completely understood.

Nerve impulses travel along nerve fibers and combine forming **spiral ganglion,** (ganglia is plural), in the **modiolus,** deep in the centre of the bony labyrinth.

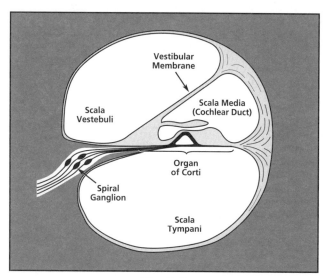

Fig. 5-7
Cross section of Cochlea

The ganglion unite, like a cable, forming the **cochlear nerve,** transmitting **electro-chemical energy.** The vestibular and cochlear nerves then become the **auditory nerve (VIII Cranial Nerve).**

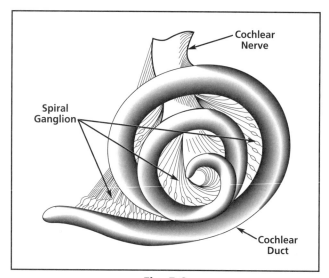

Fig. 5-8
Cochlea

Each nerve fiber can operate in only one of two ways, 'fire' or 'rest'. Any single nerve fiber cannot give a greater response to a loud sound and a lesser response to a quiet sound. It is like a light switch, on or off, NOT a dimmer switch, with varying degrees of 'on'. If it responds at all, it can only respond in one way. Unlike a muscle, the auditory nerve or its fibers cannot be exercised or strengthened.

RETROCOCHLEAR

The Auditory Nerve (VIII Cranial Nerve) consists of 30,000 neural fibers (neurons), with 95% of these fibers connecting to the inner hair cells, and 5% to the outer hair cells.

These neurons are **afferent fibers.** They transmit from the cochlea to the brain. **Efferent fibers** travel from the brain to the cochlea. The function of efferent fibers is not known.

The Auditory nerve is frequency oriented, like the cochlea. High frequencies form the outside of the 'cable,' and low frequencies, the inner core.

ASCENDING AUDITORY PATHWAYS

The cochlear nerve and vestibular nerve unite, forming the Auditory Nerve, (VIII Cranial Nerve). They leave the modialus, along with the Facial Nerve, (VII Cranial Nerve), through an opening in the bone, the **internal auditory meatus.**

Each fiber is insulated effectively from its neighboring fiber as it ascends the auditory pathways on the way to the brain. The brain is also the **cerebral cortex, temporal lobe,** and **auditory cortex.** Cortex is singular, cortices is plural.

Collections of nerve fibers in the cochlea are ganglia, (ganglion is singular). When they leave the cochlea and become part of the **Central Nervous System (CNS),** they are **nuclei,** (nucleus is singular).

Nerve fibers transfer their electrical current from one nerve fiber to another by chemical transmitters. These specialized transfer points, relay stations, or way stations, are **synaptic junctions or synapses.**

Nerve fibers can branch and take more than one path. They can decussate, (cross over to the opposite or contralateral pathway), or remain on the ipsilateral (same side) pathway. They can also branch out to join other systems, Cranial Nerves, or peripheral parts of the auditory system.

By now, it is fairly clear that the ear does not hear and understand speech. The ear transmits frequencies and intensities to the brain. The brain translates these frequencies and intensities into something meaningful, speech, noise, music, etc..

More auditory fibers cross over to the contralateral pathway than stay on the same side. **Speech heard in the right ear is processed in the left hemisphere.** This hemisphere has cerebral dominance.

Is hearing with two ears better that hearing with one ear? The following are some points to ponder.

'Far-ear' effect, or, the head shadow effect. Listen with one ear only, when the source of the sound is on the opposite side of the head. Sound travels around and over the head in order to be heard. The average level of speech is reduced by about 6 dB, and the high frequencies are reduced by about 15 dB.

Binaural squelch effect. Background noise does not mask out speech as easily when both ears hear equally. The **signal-to-noise ratio improves** because of binaural squelch, but cannot occur if the ears are not balanced. A hearing loss on only one ear, or a hearing loss on both ears with only one hearing instrument, does not have the advantage of binaural squelch.

Binaural fusion. This is a combination of similar, but not identical, signals at the two ears. Present low frequency information to one ear and high frequency information to the other, slightly delayed. You hear a high and a low frequency signal. Present low and high frequency information, simultaneously. You hear one combined tone. This is the effect of binaural fusion.

Binaural summation. The apparent loudness of a sound increases 6 to 10 dB when both ears hear together, compared to only one ear hearing the sound. Binaural thresholds are also lower than either ear alone.

Binaural localization. The ability to pinpoint the source of a sound, using differences in loudness, and in time of arrival of a sound between the two ears.

Location of a sound cannot occur in all directions when hearing with one ear. The sound appears to be on the 'hearing side'. Sound from the other side appears farther away, or on the hearing side, when it is actually on the 'bad' side.

Sound localization is reduced or lost when there is a lesion (wound or damage resulting from disease) in the brainstem or midbrain.

None of these effects happen with the use of one ear only.

HOW TO PRONOUNCE THE
TECHNICAL TERMS USED IN THIS LESSON

Afferent	af' er-ent	Octave	ok' tiv
Basilar	bas' i-lar	Osseous	ah-see' us
Cochlea	kok' le-ah	Perilymph	per' i-limf
Corti	kor'-te	Reissner's	ris' nerz
Efferent	ef' er-ent	Saccule	sak' ul
Endolymph	en' do-limf	Scala	sca' la
Ganglion	gang' le-on	Tectorial	tek-tor' e-l
Helicotrema	hel" i-ko-tre' mah	Temporal	tem-pur´ 'l
Labyrinth	lab' i-rinth	Tonotopic	ton" o-top' ik
Lamina	lam' i-nah	Tympani	tim-pan' e
Membranous	mem' bra-nus	Utricle	u' tre-k'l
Modiolus	mo-di' o-lus	Vestibuli	ves-tib' u-le

SENSORINEURAL, CENTRAL, NON-ORGANIC

Conductive disorders are treated by a variety of medical and surgical techniques. A hearing instrument compensates for a conductive hearing loss relatively easily. Usually, increased amplification in the appropriate frequency range is all that is necessary, as the understanding of speech is not affected.

A **sensorineural loss** is caused by damage or a disorder of the **inner ear**, or of the **auditory nerve,** nerve fibers going from the inner ear to the brain stem. Older terms for a sensorineural hearing loss were 'nerve loss' or 'perceptive loss'.

A hearing loss involving the inner ear or auditory nerve is more difficult, and often impossible to treat medically. Amplification cannot satisfactorily compensate for some sensorineural hearing losses when damage or degeneration of the organ of Corti, or auditory nerve fibers is extensive.

Most individuals with sensorineural hearing loss, find that a properly fitted hearing instrument is their principal or sole means to improved hearing. Often, speechreading (lipreading), and auditory training, combine visual and auditory clues for a more successful fitting.

The higher frequencies are usually affected in sensorineural loss. A person has difficulty in hearing high frequency consonants like **f, th,** and **s.** This person cannot hear the difference between the words thin, fin, pin, shin, sin, skin. The person may also fail to hear a high pitched doorbell, a telephone ringing or the signal lights in the car.

Difficulty in speech discrimination, the understanding of speech, usually accompanies a sensorineural loss. The individual believes that 'everyone mumbles' or that 'people don't speak as clearly as they used to'.

A person with a moderate sensorineural loss speaks in a loud voice. The voice does not sound normal, unless speaking loudly. The individual does not hear their own voice well through bone conduction. Other voices also become 'wiped out' very quickly in the presence of background noise.

A person with a conductive hearing loss hears their own voice well through bone conduction, and often speaks quietly. They may speak too softly in noisy situations, as the noise is not as loud to them. A person with normal hearing raises their voice to hear over the background noise.

ORGANIC HEARING LOSS

Organic disorders involve physical damage to the hearing mechanism, neural pathways or the brain.

Recruitment is characteristic of many sensorineural cochlear losses. Recruitment occurs when a small increase in sound intensity results in a rapid increase in apparent loudness. A person with recruitment may barely be able to hear a sound of moderate intensity, but a sound of slightly greater intensity seems unbearably loud. No recruitment is present if damage is to the VIII Nerve.

Tinnitus is often present in combination with sensorineural hearing losses, and usually precedes it. It is described as a high frequency ringing or buzzing noise. The noise is often isolated at the frequency with the greatest drop on the audiogram, or the lowest point on the audiogram.

Tinnitus can be heard in one ear only, usually the ear with the greatest loss. It may be present in the other ear too, but is not noticed until the tinnitus is reduced on the loudest side. Amplification with an instrument often reduces or eliminates the tinnitus. If only one ear is amplified, tinnitus may become noticeable on the unaided ear. A hearing instrument is not a cure for tinnitus. The tinnitus returns when the hearing instrument is removed.

Tinnitus can also be heard in the center of the head if it originates in both cochleas at the same pitch and loudness. Central tinnitus, also heard in the head, is not relieved by hearing instrument use, and is often associated with head trauma.

Objective tinnitus is most commonly related to middle ear, or head and neck anatomy problems. This type of tinnitus can be heard by others, and is not reduced with amplification.

Vertigo is a hallucination of movement, arising from problems within the vestibular portion of the inner ear. The world spins about the client, or, the client feels that there is moving in space. Dizziness is a giddy or swimming sensation, and is not vertigo.

Any disorder, tumor, infection or trauma causing a unilateral decrease in vestibular function may cause vertigo.

Vertigo is common in Menieres' syndrome, and in central disorders such as epilepsy, multiple sclerosis, strokes, tumors, i.e., acoustic neuroma (VIII Nerve tumor), and anemia.

Acoustic Trauma also causes sensorineural loss. The inner ear is traumatized by exposure to a single very loud sound, explosion, or high noise levels for a long time. Often, in acoustic trauma, the hearing loss is greater on the side of the noise or explosion. The head protects the opposite ear to some degree. This type of loss usually results in degeneration of the Organ of Corti.

Noise induced hearing loss is a sensorineural loss resulting from exposure to high noise levels. The exposure may be work related, or recreational. Some of the terms used are 'boilermaker's ears' or 'tractor ears'.

Industry is much more aware of the problems created by noisy work environments. Hearing conservation and use of ear protection is mandatory in the workplace. Regular hearing tests are conducted to establish the thresholds of employees. Hearing protection is worn for the protection of the employee. Periodic hearing tests detect changes that are warning signs.

Temporary Threshold Shift (TTS), also known as **auditory fatigue,** is a reversible drop in hearing thresholds from noise exposure. It becomes a **Permanent threshold shift (PTS),** with a degeneration of the Organ of Corti, if no action is taken to protect the ears from noise.

Presbycusis is a common type of sensorineural loss. Presbycusis simply means hearing loss resulting from, or associated with, increasing age.

There are four basic types of presbycusis: sensory, central, metabolic and mechanical.

1. **Sensory** hearing loss involves the hair cells. Clients exhibit an abrupt high frequency loss.

2. **Central** hearing loss creates a mild loss, with gradual loss in the high frequencies, usually from ganglion cell loss. They have **phonemic regression**, meaning poor discrimination, for such a small amount of loss, common in patients with arteriosclerosis.

3. **Metabolic** hearing loss usually causes a defect in the chemical composition of endolymph, because of atrophy, (drying up), in the stria vascularis. It is a slowly progressive, flat hearing loss.

4. **Mechanical** hearing loss results from a change in the stiffness or compliance of the basilar membrane, or fixation of the stapes. It is a slowly progressing loss, with sharp changes in the high frequencies.

Toxins, Poisons and Drugs of many kinds affect hearing and cause a sensorineural hearing loss.

Toxins are produced by viral infections. Such diseases as whooping cough, measles, influenza, scarlet fever, mumps, diphtheria, meningitis, encephalitis, chicken pox and viral pneumonia can wreak havoc with the inner ear. These sensorineural losses are usually bilateral (both ears). There are some unilateral losses, mainly from mumps. Toxins enter the endolymph fluid through the stria vascularis.

Poisons include carbon monoxide, lead, mercury, gold, arsenic, tobacco and alcohol. Each have an effect on the inner ear.

Ototoxic drugs that cause sensorineural loss include quinine, streptomycin, neomycin and kanamycin. Neomycin is often an ingredient in eardrops. The product label will state that use is contraindicated if there is a perforation in the tympanic membrane.

Ototoxic drugs are given as antibiotics. The suspected site for damage by ototoxic drugs is the spiral ganglion.

Even common drugs, like aspirin, can cause a temporary threshold shift and tinnitus, although this is reversible when the use of aspirin is discontinued. Many patients with arthritis rely heavily on aspirin.

Congenital sensorineural loss means a loss which was present at birth. There are two types, genetic or inherited, and non-genetic or acquired. A mother, who is exposed to infections, like German measles or influenza, early in the pregnancy, can have an infant with non-genetic loss. The loss is usually bilateral, with a flat or basin shaped audiogram and good discrimination.

Sudden deafness is caused by a vascular occlusion, virus, or rupture of the round window membrane.

It requires immediate attention, and is generally unilateral. The loss is usually permanent, although some people recover their hearing without treatment.

Meniere's syndrome, sometimes called **endolymphatic hydrops,** is an excess of endolymph fluid. This sensori-neural loss is a disorder of the entire inner ear, not just the cochlea. The cause is still not well understood. Symptoms include the triad of vertigo, tinnitus and hearing loss.

Tumors. The most common is an acoustic neuroma (VIII Nerve tumor), which develops just outside the internal auditory meatus. It usually involves the vestibular and facial nerves as well. Symptoms include vertigo, tinnitus, facial paralysis, and unilateral hearing loss. A characteristic feature is the inability to understand speech. Removal of the tumor often leaves a dead ear. If a tumor is located in the 'association areas' of the cerebral cortex, the symptoms may be very vague.

Oval window fistula is a rupture of the stapes footplate, or of the annular ring, with a loss of perilymph fluid. It is caused by a trauma, or a sudden increase of intra-cochlear pressure.

Round window fistula occurs as a result of a direct trauma, barotrauma (changes in barometric pressure while diving or flying), or increased perilymph pressures.

Labyrinthitis is an inflammation or infection of the inner ear. It spreads from otitis media in the middle ear, invades the inner ear through the round window, the mastoid, or the meninges (a membrane that covers the brain). It can be serous, causing dysfunction by chemical toxins, or suppurative, creating a rapid destruction of the cochlea.

Temporal bone trauma, a fracture of the temporal bone, results from automobile accidents or blows to the head. Some fractures are visible on the eardrum, itself.

Central deafness occurs through damage or disorders within the brain or brainstem. It can be caused by

1. A tumor or abscess

2. Syphilis

3. Arteriosclerosis

4. Multiple sclerosis

5. Rh incompatibility

6. Cerebral Vascular Accidents (CVA's)

   a. Brain Hemorrhage

   b. Strokes

   c. Gunshot wounds

   d. Skull fractures

7. Lack of oxygen to the brain

   a. Drowning

   b. Carbon monoxide Poisoning

When this occurs, there are defective speech and language skills. The hemisphere that is dominant for speech is involved, usually the left.

Words used to describe this communication problem are **aphasia,** both receptive and expressive, and central or verbal **dysacusis.** The use of terms is not consistent. This is a neurological involvement, rather than something wrong with any part of the ear. Some nerve pathways or association areas may be affected.

NON-ORGANIC HEARING LOSS

Individuals believe that they have a hearing loss when there is nothing physically wrong with their hearing. These individuals are not malingering (faking), they are firmly convinced that they cannot hear well. Sometimes, they cannot hear at all. This type of loss is a **psychogenic or functional loss,** referred to as **hysterical or conversion deafness.** It occurs at any age; emotional stress or tension may be the cause.

Another category of non-organic loss is where a person purposefully pretends to have a hearing loss, usually for financial gain. The individual knows there is no true hearing loss. This person is a malingerer.

Anyone with a non-organic hearing loss may have some true hearing loss, or organic loss. The additional non-organic loss, on top of the true hearing loss, is **psychogenic overlay,** or a **functional overlay.**

In young children, the difference between a true hearing loss, nonorganic hearing loss, mental retardation, childhood aphasia, or a combination of these, is difficult to determine. This requires lengthy observation, testing and medical intervention.

HOW TO PRONOUNCE THE
TECHNICAL TERMS USED IN THIS LESSON

Aphasia	ah-fa´ ze-ah
Arteriosclerosis	ar-te˝ re-o-skle̬-ro´ sis
Congenital	kon-jen´ i-tal
Dysacusis	dis˝ ah-ku´ sis
Encephalitis	en-sef˝ ah-li´ tis
Endolymphatic hydrops	en˝ do-lim-fat´ ik hi´ drops
Hemorrhage	hem´ uh-rij
Kanamycin	kan˝ ah-mi´ sin
Lamina	lam´ i-nah
Meniere's	men˝ e-arz´
Meningitis	men˝ in-ji´ tis
Neomycin	ne´ o-mi˝ sin
Neurological	nu-ra˝ -lah´ ji-k'l
Osseous	ah-see´ us
Ototoxic	o˝ to-tok´ sik
Presbycusis	pres˝ be-ku´ sis
Psychogenic	si˝ ko-gen´ ik
Quinine	kwi´ nin
Recruitment	re-kroot´ ment
Sensorineural	sen˝ so-re-nu´ ral
Streptomycin	strep´ to-mi˝ sin
Stria Vascularis	stri´ ah vas˝ ku-lar´ is
Tinnitus	ti-ni´ tus
Vertigo	ver´ ti-go

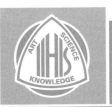

TEST INSTRUCTIONS

After you have finished reading this lesson, carefully study the selections from the **Required Reading.**

Then, look over the lesson once more to impress the important points on your memory.

When you are sure you know the lesson thoroughly, use the answer sheet in the back of the manual that corresponds to this lesson.

IMPORTANT: Place your student number on the answer sheets. Your student number appears on the inside front cover of the manual. **It must appear on your answer sheets in order for you to get credit for completion of the lesson.**

Once the answer sheet is completed, tear it out and mail to: International Institute for Hearing Instruments Studies
16880 Middlebelt Road, Suite 4, Livonia, MI 48154-3367

REQUIRED READING FOR THIS LESSON
Pages 11-21 and Pages 764-765
Hearing Instrument Science and Fitting Practices (Second Edition)
Pages 3-7
Introduction to the Auditory System

TEST QUESTIONS

1. **The adult ear canal:**
    a. is usually straight
    b. curves like a vertical figure "S"
    c. rises upward and forward, then descends to the drum
    d. descends downward, then backward toward the drum

2. **The isthmus is:**
    a. another name for the aperture
    b. located at the second bend of the canal
    c. where the canal narrows to enter the temporal bone
    d. the area between the first and second bend

3. **The pinna and the external canal together:**
    a. gather and reinforce acoustical signals
    b. with the irregular shape of the auricle, cause increases and decreases
       at different frequencies as the sound arrives at the ear
    c. forms a resonating tube
    d. all of the above

4. **The average resonant frequency of the ear canal plus concha is:**
   a. 1500 Hz
   b. 2700 Hz
   c. 3500 Hz
   d. 1000 Hz

5. **The dividing line between the external ear and the middle ear is the:**
   a. malleus
   b. Eustachian tube
   c. oval window
   d. tympanic membrane

6. **The ear canal contains:**
   a. cilia, ceruminous glands, sebaceous glands
   b. ceruminous glands, pinna, scaffoid fossa
   c. umbo, isthmus, sebaceous glands
   d. crus, aperture, sebaceous glands

7. **The Vagus Nerve (Xth Cranial) is found:**
   a. along the bottom of the tympanic membrane
   b. along the bottom of the ear canal
   c. along the bottom of the intertragal notch
   d. at the top of the isthmus

8. **Which of the following terms is not part of the tympanic membrane?**
   a. Pars tensa
   b. crus
   c. Pars flaccida
   d. Umbo

9. **An otoscopic inspection should reveal:**
   a. an external auditory canal sloping upward and backward
   b. no vision of any ossicles
   c. a clear view of the Vagus Nerve (Xth Cranial)
   d. a view of the pearly white tympanic membrane

10. **Which of the following is a part of the pinna?**
    a. tragus
    b. intertragal notch
    c. triangular fossa
    d. all of the above

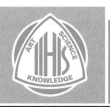
TEST INSTRUCTIONS

After you have finished reading this lesson, carefully study the selections from the **Required Reading.**

Then, look over the lesson once more to impress the important points on your memory.

When you are sure you know the lesson thoroughly, use the answer sheet in the back of the manual that corresponds to this lesson.

IMPORTANT: Place your student number on the answer sheets. Your student number appears on the inside front cover of the manual. **It must appear on your answer sheets in order for you to get credit for completion of the lesson.**

Once the answer sheet is completed, tear it out and mail to: International Institute for Hearing Instruments Studies
16880 Middlebelt Road, Suite 4, Livonia, MI 48154-3367

REQUIRED READING FOR THIS LESSON

Pages 131-133, 168, 169, 174, 796 & 797
Hearing Instrument Science and Fitting Practices (Second Edition)

Pages 30-43
Introduction to the Auditory System

TEST QUESTIONS

1. **Atresia refers to:**
   a. an active, draining ear
   b. a swollen and itching condition of the external ear canal
   c. a closure of the external auditory canal
   d. impacted wax

2. **Perforation of the eardrum can be caused by:**
   a. an infection
   b. a fracture of the temporal bone
   c. a nearby explosion
   d. all of the above

3. **The following are types of hearing loss:**
   a. conductive
   b. central
   c. sensorineural
   d. all of the above

4. **Conductive losses may be caused by:**
   a. a prolapsed canal
   b. impacted cerumen
   c. damaged hair cells
   d. (a) and (b) above

5. **Which surgical technique repairs the tympanic membrane?**
   a. cholesteaplasty
   b. lobectomy
   c. myringoplasty
   d. tympanosclerosis

6. **A cholesteatoma can be described as:**
   a. a pouch of skin filled with epithelial debris
   b. an excess of dry, brown cerumen
   c. an inflammation of the walls of the ear canal
   d. none of the above

7. **When an excess of cerumen or a blockage of cerumen is detected, the hearing aid specialist should:**
   a. proceed with ear impression
   b. refer the patient to a physician
   c. proceed with routine testing procedures
   d. remove cerumen with a Q-tip

8. **A swollen ear may be caused by:**
   a. eczema
   b. otitis externa
   c. dermatitis
   d. all of the above

9. **Tympanosclerosis may be described as:**
   a. external perforation
   b. monomeric spots
   c. calcium deposits
   d. an odorous epithelial sac

10. **A tympanic membrane perforation may cause a:**
    a. mixed loss
    b. sensorineural loss
    c. conductive loss
    d. central loss

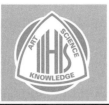
TEST INSTRUCTIONS

After you have finished reading this lesson, carefully study the selections from the **Required Reading.**

Then, look over the lesson once more to impress the important points on your memory.

When you are sure you know the lesson thoroughly, use the answer sheet in the back of the manual that corresponds to this lesson.

IMPORTANT: Place your student number on the answer sheets. Your student number appears on the inside front cover of the manual. **It must appear on your answer sheets in order for you to get credit for completion of the lesson.**

Once the answer sheet is completed, tear it out and mail to: International Institute for Hearing Instruments Studies
16880 Middlebelt Road, Suite 4, Livonia, MI 48154-3367

REQUIRED READING FOR THIS LESSON

Pages 21-27
Hearing Instrument Science and Fitting Practices (Second Edition)

Pages 8-16
Introduction to the Auditory System

TEST QUESTIONS

1. **Theoretically, the increase in sound pressure provided by the middle ear structure is about:**
   a. 12 dB
   b. 15 dB
   c. 27 dB
   d. none of the above

2. **The footplate of the stapes fits into the:**
   a. incus
   b. oval window
   c. round window
   d. incudostapedial junction

3. **A type "A" tympanogram would indicate:**
   a. possible ossicular discontinuity
   b. chronic otitis media
   c. mandatory referral
   d. normal pressure and compliance

4. **The difference in area size between the tympanic membrane and the footplate of the stapes increasing the sound pressure at the footplate is:**
   a. the transfer function or aerial ratio
   b. hydraulic energy
   c. impedance
   d. static compliance

5. **The middle ear cavity contains:**
   a. anvil, stapes and cartilage
   b. stapedius, incus, Eustachian tube and isthmus
   c. annular ligament, malleus, stapes and tensor tympani
   d. incudostapedial junction, vagus nerve, stapedius and malleus

6. **The middle ear system is often referred to as:**
   a. an impedance matching transformer
   b. attenuation method
   c. stapedial acoustic reflex
   d. fundamental transformer

7. **The middle ear cavity, as a transducer, changes energy from one form to another. The energy change is from:**
   a. mechanical energy to acoustic energy
   b. acoustic energy to mechanical energy to hydraulic energy
   c. acoustic energy to electrical energy to hydraulic energy
   d. mechanical energy to hydraulic energy to electrical energy

8. **The middle ear muscles contract, resulting in:**
   a. an acoustic reflex
   b. ossicular discontinuity
   c. increase in mechanical energy
   d. none of the above

9. **The Eustachian tube begins in the lower portion of the tympanic cavity and ends at the:**
   a. helicotrema
   b. promontory
   c. incostapedial joint
   d. nasopharynx

10. **The Eustachian tube of a child is:**
    a. straight
    b. short
    c. horizontal
    d. all of the above

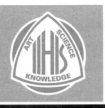

TEST INSTRUCTIONS

After you have finished reading this lesson, carefully study the selections from the **Required Reading.**

Then, look over the lesson once more to impress the important points on your memory.

When you are sure you know the lesson thoroughly, use the answer sheet in the back of the manual that corresponds to this lesson.

IMPORTANT: Place your student number on the answer sheets. Your student number appears on the inside front cover of the manual. **It must appear on your answer sheets in order for you to get credit for completion of the lesson.**

Once the answer sheet is completed, tear it out and mail to: International Institute for Hearing Instruments Studies
16880 Middlebelt Road, Suite 4, Livonia, MI 48154-3367

REQUIRED READING FOR THIS LESSON

Pages 23, 168-172
Hearing Instrument Science and Fitting Practices (Second Edition)

TEST QUESTIONS

1. **A cholesteatoma:**
   a. occurs in the middle ear
   b. may perforate the eardrum
   c. is usually accompanied by a constant odorous discharge
   d. all of the above

2. **Changes in either stiffness or mass occur when the normal middle ear function is altered by disease or trauma causing:**
   a. a swelling and/or redness in the external canal
   b. a feeling of stuffiness or a complaint of hearing in a barrel
   c. a feeling of itching deep within the ear
   d. a decrease in acoustic feedback

3. **Otosclerosis:**
   a. occurs more often in women than men
   b. occurs more often in Caucasians than other races
   c. appears to be inherited
   d. all of the above

4. **Most dysfunctions of the outer or middle ear cause a:**
   a. mixed loss
   b. conductive loss
   c. sensory loss
   d. neural loss

5. **Otitis media may occur with:**
   a. spongy changes in the bony capsule
   b. fluid in the middle ear
   c. osteoarthritis
   d. tinnitus

6. **A plastic or steel strut replaces the stapes during a:**
   a. stapedectomy
   b. stapes mobilization
   c. fenestration
   d. none of the above

7. **Treatment for chronic otitis media may include:**
   a. antibiotics
   b. inflation of the Eustachian tube
   c. myringotomy
   d. all of the above

8. **A radical mastiodectomy includes removal of:**
   a. malleus, incus and tympanic membrane
   b. tympanic membrane, malleus and Eustachian tube
   c. ossicular chain and Eustachian tube
   d. ossicular chain, mastoid

9. **The ossicular chain is supported and suspended by:**
   a. muscles only
   b. ligaments, stapedius and promontory
   c. stapedius, tensor tympani and ligaments
   d. anvil, stapedius and ligaments

10. **The ear, due to its physical characteristics, enhances which frequencies?**
    a. 250-1,000 Hz
    b. 2,000-5,000 Hz
    c. 1,000-2,000 Hz
    d. 4,000-6,000 Hz

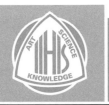
TEST INSTRUCTIONS

After you have finished reading this lesson, carefully study the selections from the **Required Reading.**

Then, look over the lesson once more to impress the important points on your memory.

When you are sure you know the lesson thoroughly, use the answer sheet in the back of the manual that corresponds to this lesson.

IMPORTANT: Place your student number on the answer sheets. Your student number appears on the inside front cover of the manual. **It must appear on your answer sheets in order for you to get credit for completion of the lesson.**

Once the answer sheet is completed, tear it out and mail to: International Institute for Hearing Instruments Studies
16880 Middlebelt Road, Suite 4, Livonia, MI 48154-3367

REQUIRED READING FOR THIS LESSON

Pages 29-41
Hearing Instrument Science and Fitting Practices (Second Edition)

Pages 10-18
Introduction to the Auditory System

TEST QUESTIONS

1. **In a cross section of the cochlea, the minimum number of rows of hair cells you can see is:**
    a. 6
    b. 5
    c. 4
    d. 3

2. **The total number of neural fibers or neurons in the human auditory nerve is about:**
    a. 10,000
    b. 20,000
    c. 30,000
    d. 40,000

3. **The basilar membrane separates:**
    a. the scala media and the scala vestibuli
    b. the scala vestibuli and the scala tympani
    c. the scala media and the scala tympani
    d. the scala tympani and the semi-circular canals

4. **The scala tympani is filled with:**
   a. strialymph
   b. perilymph
   c. endolymph
   d. cortilymph

5. **The base of the cochlea;**
   a. begins at the oval window
   b. is at the inner tip
   c. consists of low frequency sounds
   d. is wider than the apex

6. **The fibers of the auditory nerve, at the point of maximum stimulation of the basilar membrane, discharge and recover at a rate of approximately:**
   a. up to 1Khz identical to the stimulus frequency
   b. 3,000 times or cycles/sec
   c. 500 times or cycles/sec
   d. 250 times or cycles/sec

7. **The cochlea, acting as a frequency analyzer, distributes acoustic stimuli to places along the basilar membranes according to frequency. This forms the basis of a hypothesis called the:**
   a. critical band theory
   b. square wave theory
   c. place theory
   d. Fourier theory

8. **Each of the semi-circular canals:**
   a. are oriented at 90° to one another
   b. contain perilymph and endolymph
   c. detect positioning and balance
   d. all of the above

9. **Collections of nerve fibers are called:**
   a. ganglia and synapses
   b. membrane and nuclei
   c. ganglia and nuclei
   d. ganglia and cortex

10. **Afferent fibers:**
   a. transmit from the cochlea to the brain
   b. transmit from the brain to the cochlea
   c. transmit from the middle ear to the cochlea
   d. transmit from the tympanum to the brain

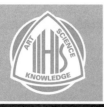
TEST INSTRUCTIONS

After you have finished reading this lesson, carefully study the selections from the **Required Reading.**

Then, look over the lesson once more to impress the important points on your memory.

When you are sure you know the lesson thoroughly, use the answer sheet in the back of the manual that corresponds to this lesson.

IMPORTANT: Place your student number on the answer sheets. Your student number appears on the inside front cover of the manual. **It must appear on your answer sheets in order for you to get credit for completion of the lesson.**

Once the answer sheet is completed, tear it out and mail to: International Institute for Hearing Instruments Studies
16880 Middlebelt Road, Suite 4, Livonia, MI 48154-3367

REQUIRED READING FOR THIS LESSON

Pages 168-174
Hearing Instrument Science and Fitting Practices (Second Edition)

TEST QUESTIONS

1. **Which of the following is a result of tissue and structure damage?**
   a. a threshold shift
   b. distortion of perception of frequencies
   c. disturbance of perception of loudness
   d. all of the above

2. **A sensorineural hearing loss is due to a disorder in the:**
   a. Eustachian tube
   b. middle ear
   c. inner ear
   d. ossicles

3. **A symptom of recruitment is:**
   a. tinnitus
   b. vertigo
   c. presbycusis
   d. intolerance for loud sounds

4. **Malingering is a category of:**
   a. presbycusis
   b. tinnitus
   c. non-organic loss
   d. sensorineural loss

5. **Meniere's syndrome consists of:**
   a. presbycusis and tinnitus
   b. noise trauma and vertigo
   c. tinnitus, vertigo and hearing loss
   d. central deafness, aphasia and vertigo

6. **An organic disorder is when there is damage to:**
   a. the hearing mechanism
   b. the neural pathways
   c. the brain
   d. all of the above

7. **Loudness recruitment:**
   a. is always present in presbycusis
   b. refers to abnormal loudness growth of clients with sensorineural hearing
   c. only applies to patients with central processing problems
   d. is medically correctable

8. **Tinnitus is:**
   a. a completely understood disorder
   b. often managed by hearing instruments or tinnitus maskers
   c. psychological in nature only
   d. managed only by a labyrinthectomy

9. **A characteristic of a conductive loss is:**
   a. a soft spoken patient
   b. more affected in high frequencies than lows
   c. continual vertigo
   d. a loud talking patient

10. **Which is not a characteristic of a sensorineural loss?**
    a. difficulty understanding high frequency consonant sounds
    b. recruitment
    c. hearing better in noise than in quiet
    d. tinnitus

INTERNATIONAL INSTITUTE FOR HEARING INSTRUMENTS STUDIES

DISTANCE LEARNING for Professionals in HEARING HEALTH SCIENCES

IIHIS

Unit II - Audiometric Testing

CONTENTS

The lessons in this unit cover Audiometric testing, which includes pure tone air and bone conductions tests; masking procedures; tone decay testing; audiogram interpretation and tests involving speech... all measured in Hearing Threshold Level, abbreviated HTL, or HL, and Tympanometry.

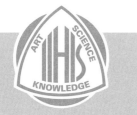

Published by
International Institute for Hearing Instruments Studies
Educational Division of International Hearing Society

IN NORMAL EARS, there are two possible routes for the sound to travel. One route uses **air conduction,** the other, **bone conduction.**

IN AIR CONDUCTION, the auricle collects and funnels sound waves in the air around us into the external auditory canal, then to the eardrum. (**Acoustic energy**). The eardrum vibrates at the same rate, and in response to, the sound waves which strike it, similar to the bass drum in an orchestra. The drum vibrates and makes the same sound, no matter what strikes it.

The difference between the eardrum and the bass drum is the eardrum stops vibrating as soon as sound ceases. The bass drum continues to vibrate, to some extent, after it has been struck.

The eardrum attaches to the malleus in the middle ear. The malleus couples to the incus, and the incus to the stapes. A ligament seals the stapes footplate in the oval window. The eardrum transmits vibrations through the tiny ossicular chain to the oval window. (**Mechanical energy**). The ossicular chain provides an effective way of converting air vibrations to fluid vibrations. It also serves a protective function for loud, low frequency sounds.

The stapes vibrates in the oval window. This sets the fluids of the inner ear in motion, creating a 'shearing action' on the hair cells imbedded in the tectorial membrane. (**Hydraulic energy**).

The hair cells respond by creating nerve impulses to the spiral ganglion. (**Electrical energy**). These impulses proceed from the modiolus to the brain. (**Chemical energy**).

Air conduction involves the transmission of sound waves from air through bones to fluid. The usual route of sound to the inner ear is by air conduction.

Sound can also arrive at the inner ear by bone conduction. The skull vibrates as a result of acoustic stimulation.

These vibrations by-pass the external and middle ear, directly stimulating the fluids of the inner ear.

IN BONE CONDUCTION, sound waves in the air strike the skull, and transmit vibrations through the bones to the fluid-filled cochlea.

Anyone who can hear at all hears partly by air conduction and partly by bone conduction. A person with a normal hearing mechanism hears almost entirely by air conduction, except for his own voice, which is a combination of bone and air conduction. When most people hear a recording of their own voice for the first time, they rarely recognize themselves. They are hearing their voice through air conduction only, instead of the usual combination of air and bone conduction.

To demonstrate bone conduction, just scratch your head. You hear the scratching noise mostly by bone conduction. Now scratch the back of your hand. The sound you hear is generated by air conduction.

An **Air-Bone Gap** is the name of the difference in sensitivity between bone conduction and air conduction. **An air-bone gap is always better hearing by bone conduction than by air conduction, never the reverse.** We normally hear better by air conduction than bone conduction. An air-bone gap indicates impairment to the conductive portion of the hearing mechanism.

In rare cases, an individual's eardrum and ossicular chain are missing. Air conduction through the ear canal and middle ear cavity reaches the oval and round windows at the same time. Some or all of the sound is cancelled, creating a greater loss of hearing sensitivity.

FREQUENCY RANGE

The normal ear can respond to a range of frequencies from about **20 Hz to 20,000 Hz.** Some authorities give slightly different figures for this range, with the lower limit between 12 to 20 Hz, and the upper limit between 12,000 to 20,000 Hz.

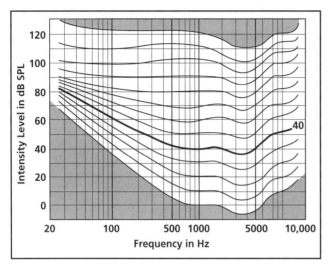

Fig. 7-1 Equal Loudness Contours

The human ear cannot hear equally well at all frequencies. In general, it is most sensitive to sounds between 3,000 and 4,000 Hz. In Figure 7-1 above, the graph is expressed in dB SPL (Sound Pressure Level). It shows how sensitivity varies at different frequencies. The quietest sounds the best human ears can hear are shown by the lowest curved line in the illustration.

The horizontal scale, along the bottom of the graph, is a logarithmic scale. The number at the extreme left is 20 Hz. The eight vertical unevenly spaced lines between 100 and 1000 Hz represent, from left to right: 200, 300, 400, 500, 600, 700, 800, and 900 Hz. The values for the eight lines between 1000 and 10,000 Hz are 2000, 3000, 4000, 5000, 6000, 7000, 8000, and 9000 Hz.

The curved lines are **equal loudness contours** or **phon lines.** A phon measures equal loudness balance at different frequencies. At 1000 Hz, phons and decibels correspond. To determine how many phons a sound of another frequency is, the other frequency is compared to the loudness of the 1000 Hz tone. Each curved line connects tones of different frequencies. Although the apparent loudness of each tone on a line is the same, the intensity required to produce this apparent loudness is different.

On the graph of equal loudness contours, take a look at the contour marked 40. **By definition, 40 phons at 1000 Hz equals 40 dB SPL.** The intensity at 100 Hz increases to 60 dB SPL to be the loudness unit of 40 phons - as loud as the 40 dB SPL tone at 1000 Hz. In other words, a tone at 1000 Hz of 40 dB intensity, sounds equal in volume to a tone at 100 Hz of 60 dB intensity. More intensity is needed in the lower frequency to make it sound equally loud.

Increasing a 1000 Hz tone by 10 dB produces an equal loudness contour at 100 Hz only about 5 dB louder, and at 30 Hz only about a 2 dB increase occurs. Once the low frequency sound is loud enough to hear, it grows louder more quickly than a 1000 Hz tone. The lowest equal loudness curve shows 0 dB at 1000 Hz, but takes an intensity of about 65 dB to even be heard at 30 Hz.

The graph shows that our 'pattern' of hearing is not the same at all contour lines. Each contour line has a slightly different shape. The bottom lines are more 'curvy'. The lines gradually flatten out as the intensity increases. This is an important characteristic of the human ear. A comfortable listening level consists of equal intensities at each frequency.

We use the terms **low tone** and **high tone** in describing frequencies, with the dividing line at 1000 Hz.

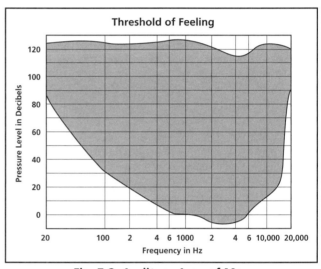

Fig. 7-2 Auditory Area of Man

The **area of effective hearing,** shown in the shaded area of Figure 7-2, occupies the equal loudness contours portion of the preceding diagram. On this diagram, you can find the **frequency range** for any given intensity level. Read the frequency range going across the graph. For example, at a level of 20 dB, the ear responds to a frequency range of 200 Hz through 15,000 Hz.

You can also find the **intensity range** for a given frequency. The intensity range goes up the graph. For example, at 1000 Hz, the intensity range is from 0 dB to about 125 dB. This intensity range is the **dynamic range.** The upper boundary is extremely loud. Sound above this level causes discomfort, and further increase causes pain.

Although the above graphs are similar, they express two different concepts. This type of graph will become very familiar to you as **'the auditory area of man' graph.** We cannot change this auditory area, but we can increase our understanding of the hearing process by using this graph to illustrate new concepts in a different way.

A person with hearing loss could have all of the auditory area affected in some way. The range of frequencies that are important for us to achieve better communication skills is much narrower, from 125 Hz to 8000 Hz, but the intensity range remains the same as the auditory area of man. Both the frequency and intensity ranges of our patients are tested on an audiometer.

ANSI STANDARDS for AUDIOMETRIC EQUIPMENT

When you test hearing with an audiometer, you compare the hearing of your patient to an arbitrary standard level, **zero on the audiometer,** representing the level research verifies as 'normal hearing'.

The zero level is **audiometric zero.** This is not the quietest sound the best human ears can hear, nor is it where sound begins. **It is a point where normal ears can hear at every frequency.** Of course, some people can hear better than others at this point. Many audiometers measure minus 10 dB HL as well.

This level has been revised several times over the years, ASA (1951), ISO (1964) and ANSI (1969). The range of normal hearing did not change, but the methods of measuring improved. The zero reference point, set by the **American National Standards Institute (ANSI) in 1969, created an international standard.**

Audiometric zero is 0 dB HL, or 0 dB hearing level. Any volume or dB level on the audiometer is a hearing level comparison to normal ears, and must include the letters HL after the number of dB, i.e. 10 dB HL, 70 dB HL. **The identification of HL is extremely important as there are several kinds of dB.**

Your audiometer is calibrated to **ANSI standards.** The law, in most states and provinces, requires calibration periodically, usually yearly.

ANSI standards have a built-in cushion in dB SPL to convert the audiometer to 0 dB HL - the threshold of average normal ears, and, of course, this level is different at each frequency.

ANSI Standards to Convert to Audiometric Zero		
Frequency	dB SPL TDH-39 earphones	dB SPL TDH-49 & 50 earphones
125 Hz	45.0 dB	47.5 dB
250 Hz	25.5 dB	26.5 dB
500 Hz	11.5 dB	13.5 dB
750 Hz	8.0 dB	8.5 dB
1000 Hz	7.0 dB	7.5 dB
1500 Hz	6.5 dB	7.5 dB
2000 Hz	9.0 dB	11.0 dB
3000 Hz	10.0 dB	9.5 dB
4000 Hz	9.5 dB	10.5 dB
6000 Hz	15.5 dB	13.5 dB
8000 Hz	13.0 dB	13.0 dB

HEARING LOSS

Anyone who is not familiar with hearing loss assumes that it is like turning the volume on a radio lower and lower until, either you have difficulty understanding the words, or cannot hear at all. Hearing loss is far more subtle than that. A person with hearing loss usually has a different amount of loss at each frequency across the range of hearing. For example, a person may have **normal hearing** in the lower frequencies, a **moderate loss** in the middle frequencies and a **severe loss** in the higher frequencies.

In order to understand, this person wants the low frequencies unchanged, the middle frequencies a little louder, and the high frequencies very loud. Increasing the volume of the radio makes all the frequencies louder. The volume is so loud in the lower frequencies, where the hearing is normal, that it becomes intolerable. Louder does not mean clearer unless the frequencies are properly balanced.

The pattern of hearing loss varies from person to person. When fitting a hearing instrument, you must know what this loss pattern is, so you can adapt the hearing instrument to individual requirements.

The technique used to determine this pattern is **audiometry,** a procedure that measures the sensitivity of a person's hearing, **relative to the sensitivity of average normal hearing.** The results of audiometric testing determine if a person has a hearing loss, what the loss pattern is, and helps to decide some of the factors involved in fitting the hearing aid.

The otolaryngologist also uses audiometric tests to compare his patient's hearing to normal hearing. The test results assist in diagnosing hearing problems, and select appropriate subjects for surgery, medical treatment, or further diagnostic testing.

Audiometry includes testing with pure tones, both by air conduction and bone conduction, and using speech as a stimulus instead of pure tones. **An audiometer,** suitable for our purposes, is capable of pure tone testing, masking and speech tests. An audiometer designed for pure tone testing only is a screening audiometer.

THE TEST ENVIRONMENT

Ideally, every hearing test should be done in a sound controlled environment, either a sound booth or a sound treated room. In any other environment, take every precaution to ensure that the test environment is as quiet as possible. Turn off fans, unplug appliances, do whatever you can to improve the validity of test results.

AUDIOMETERS

Audiometers are made by a number of manufacturers, and vary in complexity and control layout. Controls or indicators may be dials, buttons or switches.

Every audiometer has the following:

1. **A headset,** consisting of two earphones on an adjustable band that fits over the head. Earphones are color coded, red for right ear, blue for left ear.

2. **An indicator to select the ear to be tested,** either left or right.

3. **A frequency indicator** tests the following frequencies:

125 Hz	250 Hz	500 Hz	750 Hz
1000 Hz	1500 Hz	2000 Hz	3000 Hz
4000 Hz	6000 Hz	8000 Hz	

The sound produced at each frequency is a **pure tone.**

4. **An interruptor switch** controls both
   a) **when the test tone is 'on', and**
   b) **the duration of the tone.**

5. **An indicator changes the presentation of the tone** from interrupted (normal choice), to pulsed, continuous, or warble tones.

6. **The hearing level indicator** or **attenuator** controls the volume or intensity of each tone you present. This dial measures the **volume, expressed in decibels Hearing Level, dB HL,** in five decibel steps from zero dB dB steps). **Three frequencies have limits less than 110 dB HL, - 125 Hz, 250 Hz, and 8000 Hz.**

7. **An indicator changes the audiometer function** from microphone, to air conduction, to bone conduction, or to speech testing.

8. **A microphone** helps you to communicate with the patient while the headset occludes the ears.

9. **A monitor** is important when you use a two-room test suite, a sound booth, or recorded speech tests.

10. **A bone receiver** on a headband will be discussed in bone conduction testing.

11. **A masking indicator** produces a white or other noise to isolate an ear during certain tests.

The balance of the buttons or indicators will be discussed, as required, for additional tests.

Research in the fields of acoustics and audiology constantly provide improved methods and techniques for pure tone testing. The procedures outlined in this lesson represent the current views regarding the practical aspects of fitting hearing instruments. These procedures do not necessarily apply to other types of audiometric testing, such as for research or medical diagnosis.

SEATING ARRANGEMENT

Seat your patient facing slightly away from your audiometer. You do not want the patient to observe visual clues while you test, but you want their responses visible to you.

Prior to audiometric testing, complete an otoscopic examination and case history. Have excess or impacted wax removed by a physician, if necessary.

Always start your testing procedures on the better ear. If both ears are about the same, begin testing with the right ear.

The purpose of pure tone air conduction testing is to determine the threshold of the patient at every test frequency.

Threshold is the quietest level the patient can hear the tone 50% of the time. The patient does not have to hear the tone every time, just half or more of the times that you present it.

Prior to placing earphones on the patient, remove glasses, hearing instrument, earrings, etc. Extend the headband to open it to the largest size. Move hair away from the ears. Use the red earphone on the right ear and the blue earphone on the left ear. Place the earphones over the ear so they are centered exactly over the subjects' ears. The small, round center of the earphone is directly over the concha bowl, and the tragus is not pushed inward, closing off the canal opening. While holding the earphones in place, use both thumbs to gently lower the headband securely on the head.

Some people are nervous and tense in this kind of situation. Try to put them at ease by your own relaxed and confident manner.

When the headset is on the ears, it is difficult to communicate with your patient. Shouting is not an effective method. Use the microphone.

Whenever you are about to do anything, carefully explain to the patient,

a) what you are going to do, and
b) what you want them to do, or how you want them to respond.

Instructions to your patient are extremely important and cannot be over-emphasized.

There are several ways for the patient to respond:

Raise your right hand when the tone is heard in the right ear; your left hand when the tone is in the left ear. For instance:

Please let me know when you hear the tone,
    OR
Please let me know when you think you hear the tone,
    OR
Please let me know when you are sure you hear the tone.

Depending on the instructions you give, the patient's audiogram can differ by as much as 10 dB.

Your instructions to the patient should be similar to this. "Beginning with your right ear first, you will hear a tone, a buzzing sound. I want you to raise your right hand when you think you hear the tone in your right ear, and raise your left hand when you think you hear the tone in your left ear. Please raise your hand whenever you think you hear the tone, no matter how quiet it is. Do you understand?"

A good starting level is 40 dB HL. If the patient does not respond at this level, increase in 10 dB steps until a response is heard.

1. The basic technique of pure tone testing is to present a tone to the patient, one frequency at a time, starting the presentation level where it can be heard easily.

2. Gradually decrease the presentation level (**descending technique**) by turning the hearing level dial down in **10 dB steps**, presenting the tone at each lower intensity, until the tone is no longer heard. Mentally, record the last level.

3. Raise the intensity of the tone (**ascending technique**) in **5 dB steps**, presenting the tone at each level, until it is heard again. **Threshold is the lowest point where the tone is heard 50% of the time.**

4. **Bracket** to find the exact threshold. To bracket,
   a) present the tone, decreasing the presentation level 10 dB, until the patient no longer hears it.
   b) raise the presentation level 5 dB. Present the tone again. If it is not heard, again raise the level by 5dB, presenting the tone and raising the level until the tone is heard (third time). Was it the same as the other two times?

5. Bracket as often as necessary to be sure you find the lowest level the tone is heard 50% of the time. This is threshold.

For example. Frequency is 1000 Hz. Right Ear.
Present tone at:

40 dB	Tone is heard	Descending Technique
30 dB	Tone is heard	(Down 10 dB)
20 dB	Tone is heard *	
10 dB	No response.	
15 dB	No response.	Ascending Technique
20 dB	Tone is heard *	(Up 5 dB)
10 dB	No response.	Bracketing No. 1
15 dB	No response.	(Down 10 dB, up 5 dB
		steps until heard)
20 dB	Tone is heard *	
10 dB	No response.	Bracketing No. 2
15 dB	No response.	(same as No. 1)
20 dB	Tone is heard *	

You have four responses at 20 dB, and no responses at 15 dB, although there were three opportunities to respond. The recorded threshold is 20 dB HL at 1000 Hz.

- **A rule of thumb**:
   If the response is 'Yes', drop down 10 dB,
   If no response, increase 5 dB.

You will automatically be following the proper procedure for pure tone air conduction testing, including bracketing.

When you find the threshold, record it immediately on an audiogram. Threshold is the reading, in dB HL, on the hearing level dial.

THE AUDIOGRAM

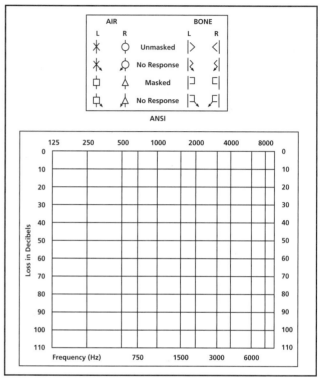

Fig. 8-1
Blank Audiogram

The vertical lines on the audiogram represent the frequencies corresponding to the audiometer frequency dial. The lowest test frequency is 125 Hz on the left of the audiogram, and the highest, 8000 Hz, on the right. **Octaves** are arranged in numerical order across the top of the audiogram.

Remember, an octave is when the higher frequency is double the lower frequency. When you double 125 Hz, then the interval between 125 Hz and 250 Hz becomes one octave. One octave from 250 Hz is 500 Hz. There are six octaves from 125 Hz to 8000 Hz.

The half-octaves are represented on the bottom of the audiogram, 750 Hz, 1500 Hz, 3000 Hz and 6000 Hz. Notice that these are also a doubling from half-octave to half-octave.

The horizontal lines on the audiogram represent the intensity in dB HL, from 0 dB HL on the top, to 110 dB HL at the bottom.

Mark threshold with a **circle 'O' in red for the right ear**, and an **'X' in blue for the left ear.** The easiest way to remember these symbols and colors is by the 'Three R's' - **Red, Right and Round.**

The symbols for air conduction are uniform worldwide, as is the color code, red for the right ear, and blue for the left.

Record the threshold on the frequency line where the frequency and the intensity in dB HL intersect.

For instance, if the patient hears a 250 Hz tone in the left ear at 25 dB HL, then draw a blue X on the 250 Hz line, half way between the 20 dB and the 30 dB lines, as in the example below.

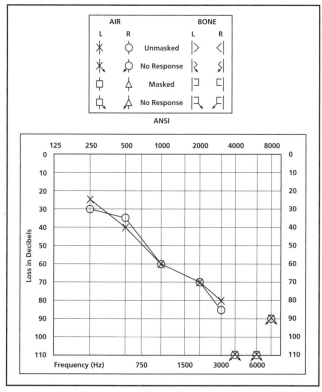

Fig. 8-2
Recording Thresholds

You might think that this patient has a 25 dB hearing loss at 250 Hz, but, more correctly, the hearing level is 25 dB HL. Normal is not the exact zero point. Normal is a range between 0 dB HL and 20 dB HL on the audiogram.

Since the patient has a threshold of 25 dB HL, the loss of sensitivity is only 5 dB if normal range is 0 - 20 dB HL. This loss of sensitivity is what 'hearing loss' means. Hearing loss is slightly less than the measured hearing threshold level.

Classification of Loss:

0 dB HL	Normal ears can hear all frequencies
0 - 20 dB	Normal range
21 - 40 dB	Mild Loss
41 - 70 dB	Moderate Loss
71 - 90 dB	Severe Loss
91 dB plus	Profound Loss

During the testing procedure, find each threshold and record it immediately on the audiogram. If you turn the hearing level dial to the test limit for that frequency, but the subject still cannot hear the tone, use an angled, downward pointing arrow to indicate that you tested this level and the tone was not heard. In Figure 8-2, this occurred at 4000 Hz, 6000 Hz and 8000 Hz. Note that the maximum level for testing at 8000 Hz is 90 dB HL, and 90 dB HL is where you place the 'no response' symbol. Connect all responses heard with a straight line for each ear. Do not connect symbols of the tones not heard.

ANSI suggests the order of presentation of frequencies be 1000, 2000, 4000, 8000, 1000, 500, 250, and 125 Hz.

Begin testing at 1000 Hz. This frequency is easy to hear and has good test, re-test reliability.

Next, test 2000 Hz, 3000 Hz / 4000 Hz / 6000 Hz / 8000 Hz

Retest 1000 Hz. This retest establishes whether the response is consistent and the instructions are understood. Response must be + or - 5 dB from the first threshold at 1000 Hz. If the threshold differs from this range, stop testing, re-instruct the patient, and re-start the test. If the threshold falls within the above range, proceed testing the lower frequencies. 500 Hz / 250 Hz.

Good hearing instrument fitting procedures require testing the intermediate, half-octave frequencies 750 Hz, 1500 Hz.

When thresholds drop from one octave to another, find out exactly where that drop occurs. For example, when a threshold at 1000 Hz is 15 dB HL, and 35 dB HL at 2000 Hz, the question arises, "Did the hearing sensitivity change at 1500 Hz, or at 2000 Hz?" This information is important in fitting a hearing instrument.

People with a noise induced hearing loss have a loss pattern that forms a 'V' notch on the audiogram. This notch occurs at 3000 Hz, 4000 Hz, or 6000 Hz. If half-octaves are not tested, this 'V' notch remains undetected.

An alternate order of frequency presentation is 1000 Hz, 500 Hz, 250 Hz, retest 1000 Hz, 2000 Hz, 3000 Hz, 4000 Hz, 6000 Hz, and 8000 Hz. Either order of presentation can be used.

Should your testing methods vary or you test in a slightly different order, consistency for each ear is imperative.

When presenting the tone, allow the tone to be on for about one second. You are not trying to trick the patient into not hearing the tone. Pressing the switch harder will not help the patient to hear the tone either, but it will give visual clues. You cannot press harder without dropping your shoulder as you press. Be sure your posture remains unchanged. Watch your body language.

Vary the pause between presentations, not the length of the tone. If the pauses are at equal intervals between presentations of the tone, your moves can be predicted. A response will be made even though a tone was not heard.

SENSATION LEVEL

When you present a tone at 40 dB HL, and the patient's threshold is 20 dB HL, the sensation level of the tone the patient hears is 20 dB SL. (40-20 =20). If you present the tone at 55 dB HL, then the sensation level is 55-20 = 35 dB SL.

You now know three kinds of dB.

1. 25 dB HTL   (Hearing Threshold Level) OR
   25 dB HL   (Hearing Level)

Both of these decibels compare the hearing of the patient to normal ears at audiometric zero, ANSI Standards.

2. 25 dB SPL (Sound Pressure Level) compares this level to where the best human ears can hear.

3. 25 dB SL (Sensation Level) - The amount of sound above the threshold of the patient, the volume the patient hears. You do not know the level in dB HL or in dB SPL unless you also know the patient's threshold.

The procedure for pure tone testing, covered in this lesson, works well for people with normal hearing or bilateral hearing loss (when the loss on both ears is approximately the same). This procedure does not apply to people who have a unilateral loss (loss on one ear only), a large threshold difference between ears, or one dead ear.

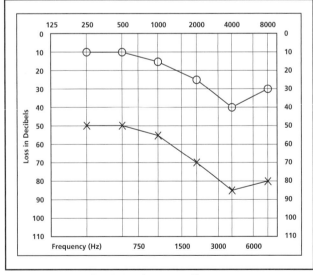

Fig. 8-3 Mirror Audiogram

MIRROR AUDIOGRAM

When using this procedure on the poorer ear, the tone becomes loud enough to cross over the head and the good ear hears the tone before the poorer ear threshold

has been found. The patient may not even be aware that the good ear responds, only that the tone is heard. The result is a 'mirror audiogram', or a 'shadow curve'. The threshold just obtained is NOT the true threshold. The point where the cross-over occurs is recorded instead.

Interaural attenuation (IA) is the loss of acoustic energy of a sound as it travels from the test ear, across the head, to the opposite ear.

Cross-over occurs when you present a sound to the test ear, but the non-test ear (other ear) hears the sound first. The cross-over level, or interaural attenuation, differs at each frequency, and varies slightly from patient to patient.

Frequency (Hz)	125	250	500	1000	2000	4000	8000
Interaural Attenuation (dB)	40	40	50	55	60	65	70

Fig. 8-4 Interaural Attenuation Levels

Rather than committing this chart to memory, a 'rule' covers all the possibilities.

Interaural attenuation (IA) for pure tone air conduction testing is 40 dB HL.

In order to test the poorer ear and find an accurate threshold, you must keep the good ear busy with another noise while testing the poorer ear. The noise that keeps the good ear busy is **masking.**

The occlusion effect is the natural increase in the loudness of a tone by bone conduction when a blockage is present. The occlusion effect is greatest at 250 Hz, about 20 dB with the type of ear cushion in common use, 15 dB at 500 Hz, reducing to 10 dB at 1000 Hz.

AUDITORY FATIGUE

Any temporary threshold shift is **auditory fatigue,** a change in the threshold of hearing as a result of continuous exposure to sound. Auditory fatigue is usually present to some degree with noise induced losses, which begin as a temporary threshold shift, and over time, becomes permanent.

Auditory fatigue also occurs when a continuous stimulus, presented at a level above threshold, appears to fade in volume until it is no longer audible.

Tone decay tests are designed to measure the auditory fatigue of the VIII Nerve.

When excess tone decay occurs, medical referral is required. This is one possible symptom of an acoustic neuroma, or VIII Nerve tumor. Other symptoms of acoustic neuroma include difficulty understanding speech, tinnitus, and vertigo. These symptoms also require medical referral.

A tone decay test is administered in the higher frequencies, using a continuous tone for a period of one minute. The recommended frequency for tone decay testing is 4000 Hz unless restricted by the upper limits of the audiometer or the hearing loss. Use 2000 Hz when restricted. Using the Olson-Noffsinger method, instruct the patient to raise the appropriate hand for as long as the tone is present, and lower it when the tone disappears.

Present a continuous 4000 Hz tone at 20 dB SL (20 dB above the patient's threshold at 4000 Hz) for one minute, or until the hand is lowered.

If the patient hears the tone for the entire minute, record the test ear and result, i.e., left tone decay negative at 4000 Hz.

If the patient ceases to hear the tone before the minute passes, then record, for example, right tone decay positive at 4000 Hz.

If decay is present, test again at a lower frequency. State both the frequencies tested and the method in your referral letter.

PURE TONE BONE CONDUCTION TESTS

LESSON 9

A pure tone air conduction test transmits sound through the outer and middle ear to the stapes footplate and then through the fluid filled cochlea.

A bone conduction test bypasses the outer and middle ear, testing the cochlea directly, by vibration to the skull. A bone conduction oscillator is used instead of earphones. Any outer or middle ear problem which causes hearing loss will be absent when testing the cochlea by bone conduction.

The definition of a conductive loss includes any blockage, breakdown, or obstruction of the outer or middle ear. An air conduction test measures the amount of hearing loss present including this blockage, breakdown or obstruction. The bone conduction test measures the cochlea directly, measuring the amount of loss causing the breakdown or blockage, the conductive component. We also find the potential hearing ability of the cochlea, the cochlear reserve.

As most conductive losses are medically correctable, bone conduction test results show the improvement medically possible in the patient's hearing without the use of a hearing instrument. The bone conduction test may also show a mixed loss, with a medically correctable portion and a portion requiring the use of a hearing instrument. Both a conductive loss and mixed loss have bone conduction thresholds better than air conduction thresholds, never the reverse. Sensorineural loss thresholds are the same for both air and bone conduction tests.

Occasionally, a bone conduction threshold is worse than the air conduction threshold. This can be due to the placement of the vibrator, the thickness of the skull, damage to a part of the skull that restricts proper vibration, or excess fat covering the bones of the skull. This phenomenom occurs most often at 500 Hz.

When bone conduction thresholds are worse than air conduction thresholds, this is **not** a cause for referral. You are testing the same cochlea.

PURPOSE

A bone conduction test determines the threshold of the cochlea directly, and establishes if a conductive component exists at any frequency in the hearing loss of the patient.

THRESHOLD

As in air conduction testing, threshold is when the patient responds to the softest tone 50% of the time. With masking, the patient must hear the threshold tone in the test ear 100% of the time.

ORDER of PRESENTATION

The order of presentation of bone conduction frequencies is the same as for air conduction testing. Begin at 1000 Hz, increasing to 2000 Hz, 4000 Hz, 500 Hz and 250 Hz. Half octaves are not tested routinely. Audiometers are not capable of bone conduction testing at 125 Hz, 6000 Hz or 8000 Hz.

AUDIOMETRIC LIMITS

The maximum limit of the audiometer for bone conduction testing is much smaller than for air conduction tests. 250 Hz has the smallest limit, 40 dB to 60 dB, with the balance of the frequencies being 65 dB to 70 dB. Especially at lower frequencies, the decibel level produced by the audiometer tactically vibrates the bone conductor.

SYMBOLS

Bone conduction symbols are not standardized. As with air conduction testing, red is used for the right ear and blue for the left ear as standard colors.

Every audiogram has a key for interpretation. Check the audiogram key to determine what the symbols represent in any textbook illustration or audiogram from other sources.

The following symbols, in common use, are recommended.

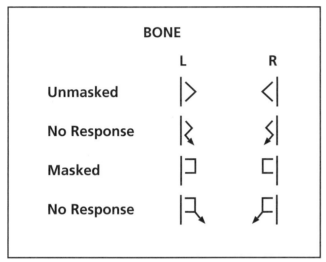

Fig. 9-1
Masking Symbols

ROOM NOISE

As with air conduction testing, room noise is critical in the lower frequencies, although the earphones attenuate some noise. Nothing covers the test ear during a bone conduction test, so room noise invalidates the test very easily. You require an extremely quiet environment during a bone conduction test because there is 0 dB interaural attenuation for pure tone bone conduction.

BONE CONDUCTION RECEIVER and HEADBAND

The bone conduction receiver is slightly concave or has a raised circle on the side lying against the skull. The headband applies pressure on the receiver, holding it tightly against the mastoid process. A loose headband gives inaccurate thresholds.

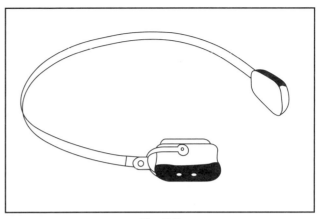

Fig. 9-2
Bone Conduction Receiver and Headband

PLACEMENT of the BONE CONDUCTION RECEIVER

After moving the patients hair aside, place the receiver on the raised bone behind the ear, the mastoid process, without the receiver touching the pinna. To find the 'magic spot' on the mastoid process, put your audiometer setting on 'bone' and 500 Hz. Have the intensity dial continuously on at 40 dB, or a level where the patient can hear it easily. Move the receiver along the mastoid process, with your patient telling you where the tone seems louder. The tone increases most around the top of the ear, about 1" back from the pinna.

Although this is the ideal location, the shape of many heads does not allow the headband to fit properly in this position. The receiver will only sit securely farther down this protruding bone.

The receiver cannot be hand held into position. It also cannot touch the ear without setting up vibrations in the ear canal. The tension of the headband must be firm for it to vibrate the bones of the skull.

PROCEDURE

When testing unmasked bone conduction, start above threshold, descend to threshold, and bracket in the same manner as for air conduction.

When you put the receiver on the right mastoid process, and complete an unmasked bone conduction test for that ear, **you do not have a bone conduction threshold for the right ear**. Interaural attenuation by bone conduction is 0 dB. You have tested the best cochlea only, and do not have any idea which ear answered for sure.

What you have accomplished can look like this:

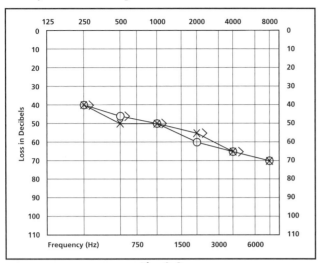

Fig. 9-3
Best Cochlea Sensorineural Response

This audiogram shows a sensorineural hearing loss with no conductive component present. The best cochlea is not better than any air conduction reading. You need no further bone conduction test, as there is no air-bone gap at any frequency.

In Figure 9-4, the audiogram shows a conductive hearing loss either the left, the right, or both ears. All you know is the best cochlea responded. You do not know which cochlea answered. You cannot assume that the best cochlea is the better ear by air conduction.

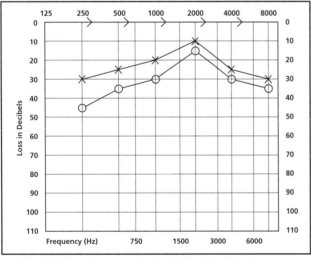

Fig. 9-4
Best Cochlea Conductive Response

This result could mean that the left ear has a sensorineural loss and you do not know about the right ear, or that the right ear has a conductive component. Remember, just because you placed the vibrator on the left mastoid, that does not mean that you tested the left ear. Whichever cochlea was better at that frequency responded.

WEBER TEST

Place the bone vibrator in the middle of the patient's forehead. Set the frequency dial to 500 Hz. and the attenuator dial to 40 dB HL, or louder if no tone is heard. Remember, bone conduction threshold maximum varies from 65 dB to 70 dB on the audiometer. Beyond this point, the sound gets quieter. Ask the patient where the tone is heard.

Three results are possible, in this order only.

1. The patient hears the tone in the ear with the greatest conductive loss at 500 Hz. (the poorer ear on the audiogram).

2. If no conductive loss is present, the patient hears the tone in the ear with the best sensorineural loss at 500 Hz, (the better ear on the audiogram).

3. If the loss at 500 Hz in both ears is identical, either sensorineural or conductive, the patient hears the tone in the center of the forehead.

You can do this test at any frequency. Conductive losses respond better in the lower frequencies. 250 Hz only has a 40 dB maximum limit, restricting your range. Sensorineural losses normally have better hearing in the lower frequencies than in the highs, making the higher frequencies more difficult to test.

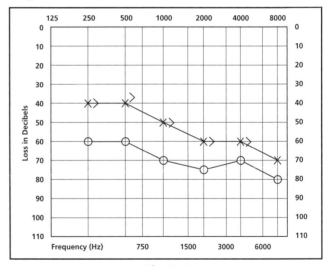

Fig. 9-5
Best Cochlea Unknown Response

As you can see from these results, in Figure 9-5, no matter where you put the bone vibrator, you are not testing a specific ear. You are either testing the occlusion effect of the biggest conductive loss, or the best cochlea in a sensorineural loss. Unmasked bone conduction tests serve a special purpose. You can test what kind of loss the patient has, but you cannot obtain a bone conduction threshold for either ear without the use of masking to isolate the non-test ear.

MASKING - PURE TONES

LESSON 10

Although the term 'masking' may be new to you, its effects occur daily. For example, You are watching TV and someone turns the dishwasher on. The TV is not loud enough for you to hear and understand over the noise of the dishwasher. The dishwasher (the masker) masks out the TV (the signal).

Lower frequency sounds mask out higher frequency sounds. Room or ambient noise has a lower frequency than conversational speech, often making speech inaudible. The **upward spread of masking** occurs when a lower frequency sound masks out a higher frequency stimulus. Higher frequency sounds do not mask out the lower frequencies as easily. In fact, some of the extremely high frequencies cannot mask another sound at all.

For our purposes, masking has two definitions.

1. Masking occurs when an unwanted sound causes a wanted sound to be inaudible.

2. Masking is required to keep a better ear busy while testing a poorer ear. The poorer ear receives the tone while the better ear hears a **controlled masking noise.**

Audiometers use several kinds of masking noise. The most common masking is **white noise,** a broad band of noise that contains equal amounts of energy in all frequencies. White noise is reasonably **effective for both pure tone and speech testing,** although listening to the noise is fatiguing for any length of time. White noise is not as efficient in the lower frequencies as it is in the higher frequencies because of the upward spread of masking.

Narrow band noise consists of a narrow range of frequencies of equal intensity. The range of frequencies making this noise changes in direct relationship to the frequency dial on the audiometer. For instance, when testing 250 Hz, the narrow band masking centers around 250 Hz: changing to 500 Hz centers the narrow band masking at 500 Hz. Narrow band noise is more effective and easily tolerated than white noise for pure tones, but is **not effective for speech tests.**

Speech Noise is **effective for speech testing**, but not effective for pure tone testing. Speech noise is white noise filtered to a low and middle frequency spectrum.

MASKING TERMINOLOGY

The test ear discriminates a signal or tone when a masking noise in the non-test ear is almost as loud, equal, or slightly louder than the tone.

Cross-over is sound that is 'heard' by the better ear when the tone or speech is presented to the poorer ear.

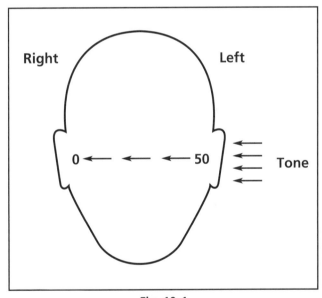

Fig. 10-1
Crossover From the Left Ear to the Right Ear
Due to Interaural Attenuation

A shadow curve or mirror audiogram occurs when the better ear 'answers' for the poorer ear. The contour of the poorer ear 'follows' the contour of the better ear with 30dB or greater hearing loss.

Interaural Attenuation (IA) is a barrier of sound transmission from one ear to the other. Interaural attenuation refers to the energy needed to transfer a sound from one ear to the other ear. This required energy is lost during transmission and not heard at the other ear. It takes about 40 decibels or more for the sound to be audible to the

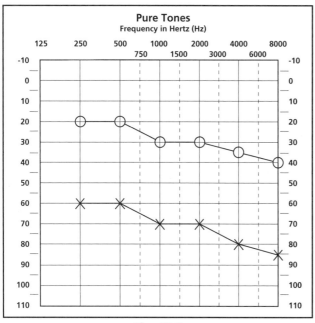

Pure Tones
Frequency in Hertz (Hz)

Fig. 10-2
Shadow Curve

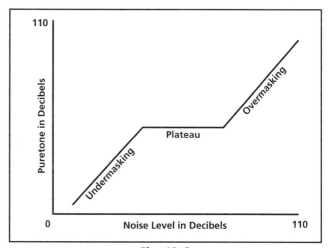

Fig. 10-3
Three Masking Shifts

opposite ear during air conduction testing. In bone conduction testing, it may take as little as 0 decibels for the sound to be audible in the opposite ear.

Effective masking (EM) eliminates cross-over from occurring. Effective masking determines how much noise is appropriate to 'cover up' or 'keep busy' the better ear or non-test ear from taking part in the test.

Undermasking occurs when the masking noise presented to the better ear is not loud enough to eliminate cross-over or interaural attenuation. The patient hears the tone in the same ear as the masking noise, the non-test ear. An increase in the masking noise causes the false threshold to shift from the non-test ear, and drop to the true threshold of the test ear (undermasking occurs more commonly in air conduction testing).

Overmasking occurs when each 10 dB increase in masking shifts the hearing threshold 10 dB or more above the plateau. Overmasking occurs more commonly in bone conduction testing.

Central Masking is a shift of 5 dB in the threshold of the test ear because of the effects of masking on the Central Nervous System (CNS). Central Masking occurs when an effective masking noise in the non-test ear isolates the test ear from cross-over or interaural attenuation, and the Central Nervous System causes the test ear threshold to be 5 dB lower than without masking.

When using a controlled masking stimulus, ideally, our noise is effective throughout the test. Undermasking allows a false, better hearing threshold, while overmasking drives the true threshold lower.

As you can see in Figure 10-3, undermasking occurs before a plateau is reached. This is where cross-over occurs. When you start on the plateau, white noise masking can be increased by 40 to 50 dB without changing the threshold of the test ear by air conduction. Verifying threshold only requires the first 20 dB of this plateau. Narrow band noise can be increased 30 to 40dB without changing threshold. Narrow band noise is 10 dB more effective than white noise.

If the masking is increased beyond the plateau, the threshold will shift because overmasking occurs. The masking noise is crossing over to the test ear and masking out the tone. If you increase the intensity of the tone, it will again be heard, but will disappear when the masking is increased.

When to Mask: Whenever the threshold of the poorer ear by air conduction exceeds the interaural attenuation of 40 dB, masking is required to obtain an accurate threshold of the poorer ear.

Masking Rule No. 1(a)

Masking is required in the better ear when the difference in air conduction thresholds between ears is 40 dB or more.

Masking Rule No. 1(b)

Whenever the masked or unmasked bone conduction threshold of the better ear is 40 dB better than the air conduction threshold of the poorer ear, mask the poorer ear thresholds by air conduction.

When in doubt mask! It is better to mask and find out that it was not required. Test results obtained without masking when there is a NEED for masking, result in improper test results and poor instrument fittings.

To determine the proper amount of masking noise and the starting level for the test tone, the following guideline is appropriate:

Instructions: Explain to the patient that the noise will be heard in the better ear and should be ignored, listening only for the test tone in the poorer ear.

Masking Noise: Start masking noise in the better ear at air conduction threshold plus 10 dB. This allows the masking noise to be audible to the better ear.

Test Tone: Start the test tone at the intensity where IA can occur, or at the unmasked threshold.

If a response is obtained with the test tone in the poorer ear, increase the masking noise by 5 dB. This procedure must be repeated three times for an increase in the masking noise by 15 dB with the test tone 'holding' and not changing it's decibel level. Once this is obtained, the test tone is a true threshold and should be recorded on the audiogram using masked response symbols.

If no response is obtained with the test tone in the poorer ear, increase the test tone until you have a response. Once a response is obtained, increase your masking noise in 5 dB increments, making certain that the response obtained in the test ear 'holds' at each of these masking noise increases. Should the test ear threshold change with an increase in masking noise level, again increase the masking noise in 5 dB increments to a maximum of 15 decibels. Once a new threshold is obtained, repeat the masking noise increases again. The test tone is a true threshold and should be marked as such on the audiogram.

Symbols used to identify that masking was used in air conduction testing are a triangle for the right ear and a square for the left ear. See following audiogram key.

Audiogram Key		
TEST PROCEDURE	**RIGHT**	**LEFT**
Air Conduction Unmasked		
Air Conduction Masked		
Bone Conduction Mastoid Unmasked		
Bone Conducton Mastoid Masked		
Bone Conduction Forehead Unmasked		
Bone Conduction Forehead Masked		
No Response Symbols		

Fig. 10-4
Pure Tone Symbols

MASKING – BONE CONDUCTION

Masking Procedures for Bone Conduction Tests: The headset of the audiometer produces the masking noise in the non-test ear. The test ear, with the bone vibrator on the mastoid process, must not be occluded in any way with the headset.

WHEN TO MASK

The plateau masking procedures also apply to bone conduction testing. Bone conduction thresholds can cross-over with 0 dB difference between ears.

Masking Rule No. 2

Mask for bone conduction when a 15 dB or more difference occurs between the bone conduction of the better ear and the air conduction of the poorer ear.

For example, you must compare the test ear air conduction threshold with the bone conducted threshold of the non-test ear at the same frequency. If the difference is greater than 10 dB (15 dB or more), masking noise must be used in the non-test ear.

Occlusion Effect: The occlusion effect may cause bone conduction thresholds to shift once headphones are placed on the head.

Again, when in doubt mask! To determine the proper amount of masking noise and the starting level for the test tone, the preceding guideline is appropriate. Symbols used to identify that masking was used in bone conduction testing are a square bracket on the left side of the frequency line on the audiogram for the right ear and a square bracket on the right side of the frequency line for the left ear (refer to figure 10-4).

Worksheet (500 Hz):

Masked Ear (Right)		Test Ear (Left)	
	Response		
Beginning Level	30	NR	5	Beginning level
	30	NR	10	
	30	NR	15	
	30	NR	20	
	30	NR	25	
	30	NR	30	
	30	NR	35	
	30	NR	40	
	30	R	45	
	35	NR	45	
	35	NR	50	
	35	R	55	
	40	R	55	
	45	R	55	
	50	R	55	

Fig. 10-5
Masking Worksheet for Fig. 10-6

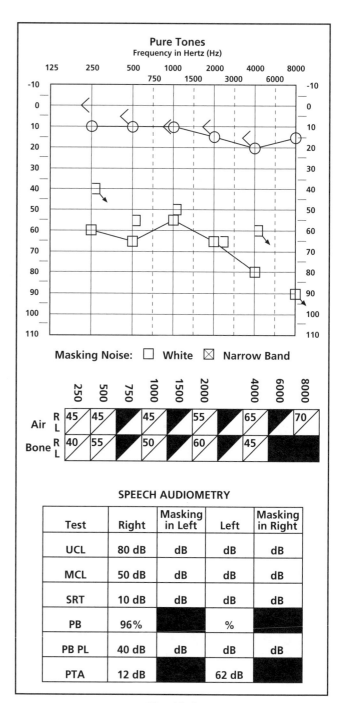

Fig. 10-6
Audiogram for Fig. 10-5

Masking Noise: ☐ White   ⊠ Narrow Band

		250	500	750	1000	1500	2000		4000	6000	8000
Air	R / L	45	45		45		55		65		70
Bone	R / L	40	55		50		60		45		

SPEECH AUDIOMETRY

Test	Right	Masking in Left	Left	Masking in Right
UCL	80 dB	dB	dB	dB
MCL	50 dB	dB	dB	dB
SRT	10 dB	dB	dB	dB
PB	96%		%	
PB PL	40 dB	dB	dB	dB
PTA	12 dB		62 dB	

DISTANCE LEARNING for Professionals in HEARING HEALTH SCIENCES

THE HEARING ANALYSIS: THE AUDIOGRAM

LESSON 11

The **diagnosis** of a person's hearing loss is the task and responsibility of the physician. The evaluation of test results - **the hearing analysis -** for hearing instrument fitting, is essential to the person who selects, fits and adjusts the hearing instrument to its maximum effectiveness.

TYPES OF LOSSES

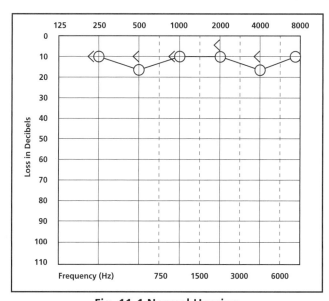

Fig. 11-1 Normal Hearing

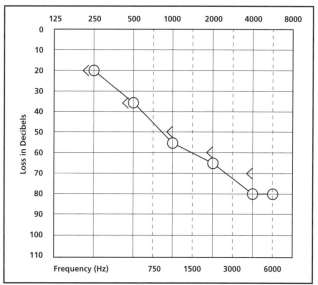

Fig. 11-2 Sensorineural Loss

NORMAL HEARING:

Fig. 11-1, above, shows a typical normal hearing audiogram for the right ear. There is no loss by either air conduction or bone conduction.

SENSORINEURAL LOSS:

A sensorineural loss, illustrated in Fig. 11-2, above, has thresholds the same by both air conduction and bone conduction. Most of the thresholds are not within normal range. There is no conductive component, the entire loss is sensorineural.

CONDUCTIVE LOSS:

A **conductive component** is the over-all difference between the air and bone thresholds, **the air-bone gap.**

A **sensorineural component** is the difference between the bone threshold and the range of normal hearing. The sensorineural threshold is the same as the loss by bone conduction. If bone conduction thresholds are not within normal limits, then some sensorineural loss has occurred.

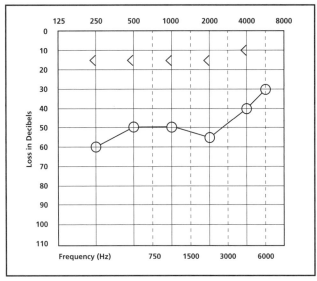

Fig. 11-3 Pure Conductive Loss

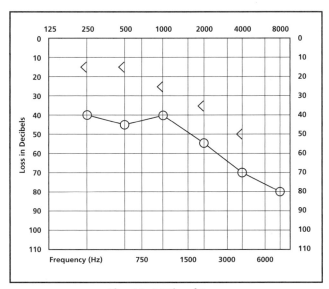

Fig. 11-4 Mixed Loss

In Fig. 11-3, all bone conduction thresholds are within normal limits, showing no sensorineural loss, with air conduction thresholds below normal limits. This is a pure conductive loss.

Remember that if the loss is purely conductive, the nerve cells in the inner ear are functioning normally, and readily respond to vibrations through the bones of the skull. The conductive mechanism of the outer or middle ear is impaired, reducing the sound before its arrival at the inner ear. **In a pure conductive loss, the bone conduction thresholds are in normal range.**

In Fig. 11-4, the bone conduction thresholds are below 20 dB HL at some or all frequencies. A sensorineural component is present in the hearing loss. This is a **mixed loss,** and exhibits both a **sensorineural component and a conductive component.** Again, the sensorineural component is the loss by bone conduction, and the conductive component is the air-bone gap. Many patients have this type of audiogram.

CLASSIFICATION of AUDIOGRAMS by SHAPE

Audiograms are classified in seven basic shapes.

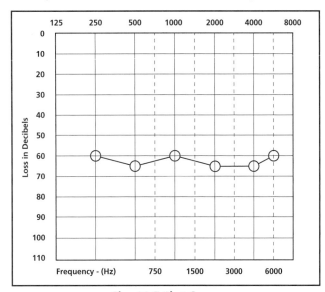

Fig. 11-5 Flat Curve

Thresholds are approximately equal at all frequencies.

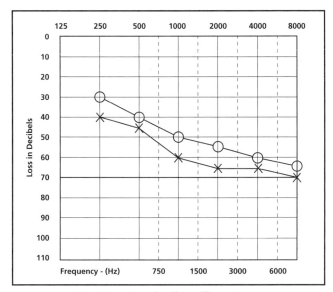

Fig. 11-6 Gradually Falling Curve

Thresholds fall off in the higher frequencies about 5 - 10 dB per octave.

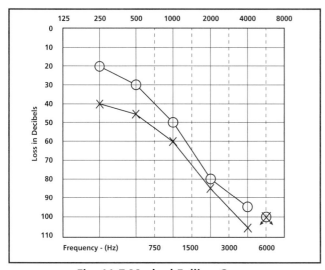

Fig. 11-7 Marked Falling Curve

Fall off is 15 - 20 dB per octave in the higher frequencies.

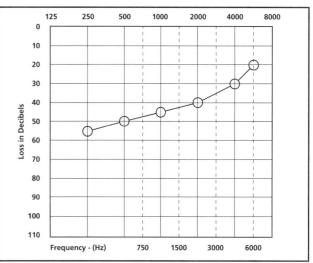

Fig. 11-8 Rising Curve or Reverse Slope

Loss decreases in higher frequencies at about 5 - 10 dB per octave.

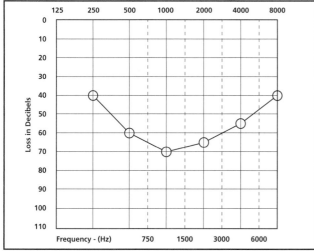

Fig. 11-9 Trough-Shaped (or Saddle Shaped) Curve, or 'cookie bite'.

Less loss at high and low frequencies than in the middle frequency region.

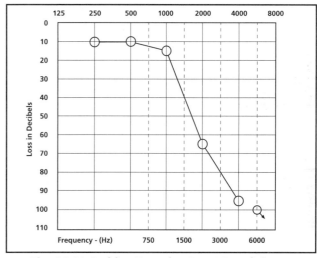

Fig. 11-10 Sudden Drop (or Steep Drop) Curve

Normal or near normal up to 1000 or 2000 Hz, with a steep drop to the next frequencies.

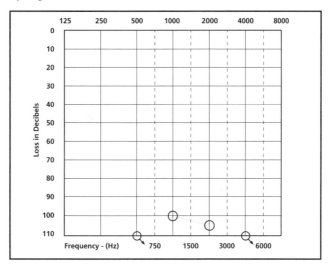

Fig. 11-11 Fragmentary Audiogram

There are small islands of hearing at one or two frequencies only.

DEGREE of HEARING LOSS

One way a hearing loss compares to the degree of difficulty in hearing is the **Pure Tone Average**. To calculate the Pure Tone Average (PTA) add the air conduction thresholds at 500 Hz, 1000 Hz, and 2000 Hz, then divide this answer by three. Your answer, in dB, is the pure tone average.

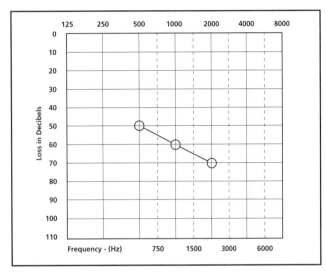

Fig. 11-12 Three Frequency PTA

For example, the audiogram above shows a loss of 50 dB at 500 Hz, 60 dB at 1000 Hz, and 70 dB at 2000 Hz. Adding the three thresholds together equals 180. Dividing by 3 produces a 60 dB pure tone average.

The pure tone average (PTA) is a good estimate of the loss for speech, and estimates the Speech Reception Threshold used in speech audiometry. This PTA is sometimes used to describe the loss in an ear. It does not accurately describe the degree of difficulty in hearing, especially when dealing with a marked falling curve or a sudden drop curve where some hearing is within normal range.

Although you can compute pure tone average for either air conduction or bone conduction, the air conduction average is customary. If the increase in loss between 500 Hz and 1000 Hz **and** between 1000 Hz and 2000 Hz is 15 - 20 dB or more, the pure tone average should be computed as follows:

Select the two frequencies that show the **least** loss, add these thresholds, and divide by two. This answer becomes the PTA.

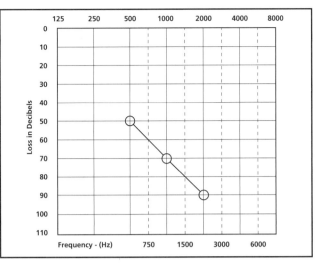

Fig. 11-13 Two Frequency PTA

For example, the audiogram above shows a loss of 50 dB at 500 Hz, 70 dB at 1000 Hz, and 90 dB at 2000 Hz. This is a severe marked falling curve.

The two frequencies which show the **least** loss are 500 Hz and 1000 Hz. Adding 50 and 70 gives you 120; dividing by two is 60 dB, the average loss.

If you use the other method, you erroneously arrive at an average loss of 70 dB.

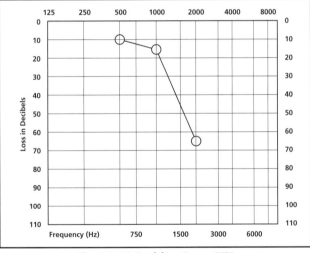

Fig. 11-14 Sudden Drop PTA

Another example, using a sudden drop curve, shows 500 Hz at 10 dB, 1000 Hz at 15 dB, and 2000 Hz at 65 dB as indicated in Figure 11-14 above. Using two frequencies with the least loss, 10 plus 15 equals 25, divided by two is 12.5 dB pure tone average. The pure tone average is totally within normal limits, yet the patient has a difficult time understanding speech.

As you can see from this example, the pure tone average does not indicate the degree of difficulty when some of the hearing is within normal range. In fact, it can be misleading in this case.

Hearing losses classify into Mild, Moderate, Severe, and Profound impairments. The following list reviews the classification of loss in Lesson 8.

Loss in dB HL	Degree of Loss
0 - 20	Normal (no loss)
21 - 40	Mild Loss
41 - 70	Moderate Loss
71 - 90	Severe Loss
91 - plus	Profound Loss

When you use the pure tone average to describe the **average hearing loss**, you have a fairly accurate description of a flat curve loss, a gradually falling curve, or a fragmentary audiogram.

Marked and sudden drop curves are more accurately described in two parts, i.e. mild to severe loss.

Signatures of Audiograms

Your signature is unique. It tells the world what your name is, and that you wrote it yourself. Audiograms have signatures, too. Information on your case history, visual clues, and other tests can all help identify signatures.

Noise Induced Loss A noise induced hearing loss forms a 'V' notch at either 3000 Hz, 4000 Hz, or 6000 Hz. The lines below the 'V' notch indicate how the notch widens over time.

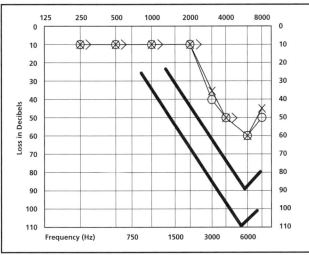

Fig. 11-15
Noise Equal on Both Ears

The thresholds on both ears can be fairly similar, an indication that the patient is surrounded by noise, like working in a noisy area or going to bars.

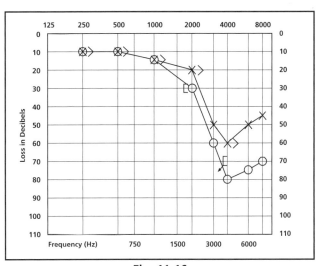

Fig. 11-16
Noise Louder on the Right

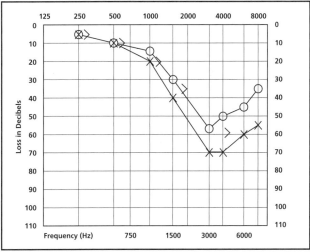

Fig. 11-17
Noise Louder on the Left

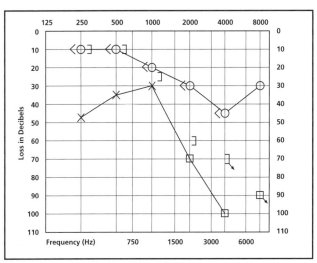

Fig. 11-18
Explosion on the Left Side

One ear slightly worse than the other occurs when noise is louder on one side. Truckers have a left threshold lower than the right, farmers look over their shoulder on the tractor, hunters hold the gun a certain way. The head protects one ear slightly.

Acoustic Trauma audiograms have a much greater separation between left and right ears, often with some conductive component. For instance, an explosion will have a far greater effect on the closer ear. Again, the head protects the other ear. High frequency tinnitus is often present in noise induced losses.

Presbycusis

Presbycusis thresholds often resemble noise induced hearing loss, without the 'V' notch.

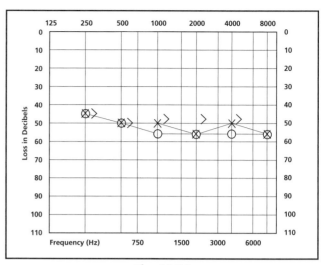

Fig. 11-21
Metabolic Presbycusis

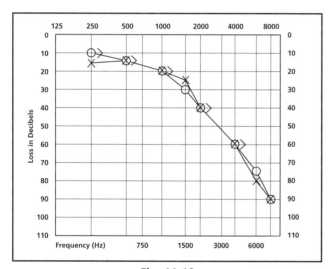

Fig. 11-19
Sensory Presbycusis

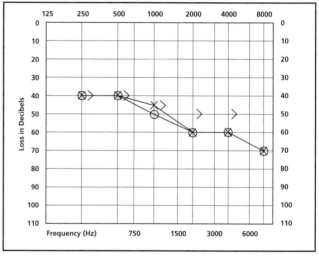

Fig. 11-22
Central Presbycusis

Review anatomy lesson 6-2 for clearer understanding of audiograms.

Central Presbycusis differs from the other three losses because of very poor speech discrimination for the small amount of hearing loss. Patients with **phonemic regression** do not find hearing instruments as successful as other presbycusis patients. Your case history may include arteriosclerosis. Difficulty answering case history questions or following your conversations also occurs. Eardrums frequently are opaque or sclerotic.

Mechanical and Metabolic Presbycusis often have a small conductive component involved, sometimes in the high frequencies only.

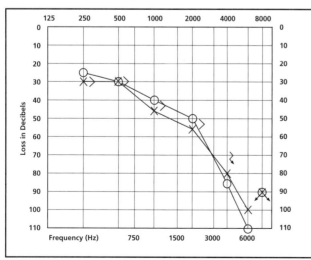

Fig. 11-20
Mechanical Presbycusis

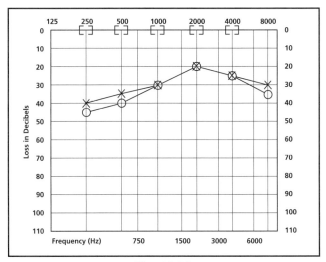

Fig. 11-23
Otitis Media

All bone conduction thresholds are in normal range, while air conduction thresholds have a reverse slope, and Type B Tympanograms.

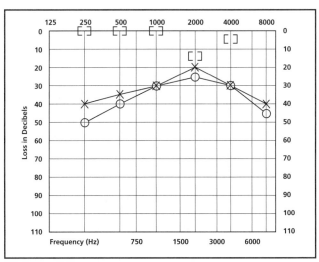

Fig. 11-24
Otosclerosis

In the early stages, this audiogram looks very similar to otitis media, with one exception. The bone conduction threshold dips at 2000 Hz. This dip is the **Carhart Notch.** Tympanograms are Type As.

If the patient has a stapedectomy, the bone conduction threshold returns to normal along with the air conduction thresholds. Without surgery, over time, the bone conduction thresholds do not stay in normal range and the loss becomes worse in the higher frequencies by both air and bone conduction.

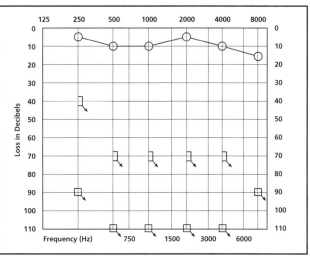

Fig. 11-25 Mumps and Sudden Deafness

Both have similar audiograms. The difference is that mumps is longstanding and sudden deafness just occurred. Refer immediately for medical evaluation. Time is very important to possible recovery.

Mumps can be unilateral or bilateral.

EUSTACHIAN TUBE DYSFUNCTION

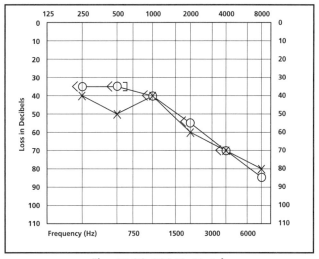

Fig. 11-26 500 Hz Notch

A small conductive notch at either 500 Hz or 1000 Hz occurs, depending on the size of the ear canal. Industrial tests on men indicate more 1000 Hz dips, although 500 Hz is more common for the general public. Tympanograms are slightly negative, but not Type C.

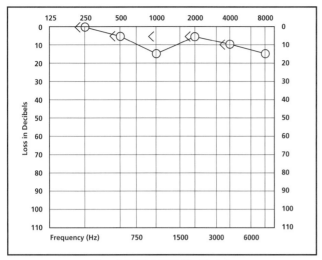

Fig. 11-27 1000 Hz Notch

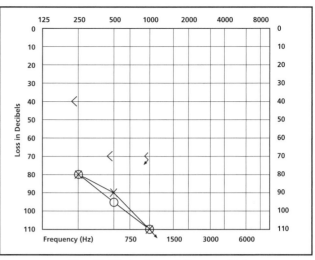

Fig. 11-29 Profound Congenital

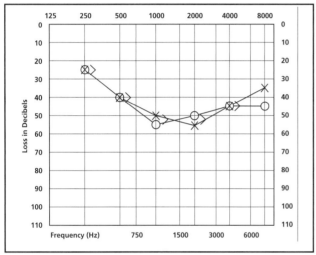

Fig. 11-28 Congenital

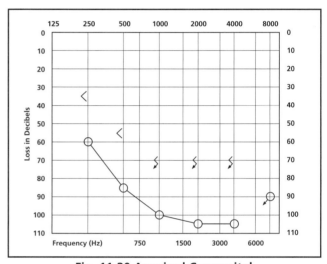

Fig. 11-30 Acquired Congenital

A congenital loss exhibits the 'cookie bite' and can drop quite quickly over time, but retains the 'cookie bite' form.

Discrimination is good. Tympanograms are Type A, with no visual clues.

A profound congenital loss may only have an island of hearing. Bone conduction thresholds often occur. Ask if the patient hears it or feels it, and if the tone changes. Usually this response is only **vibrotactile.** He feels the vibration but does not hear the tones.

Speech is affected. Discrimination is poor.

This audiogram is an acquired congenital hearing loss. When a mother has rubella in the first trimester of pregnancy, the baby's loss is acquired, but not hereditary.

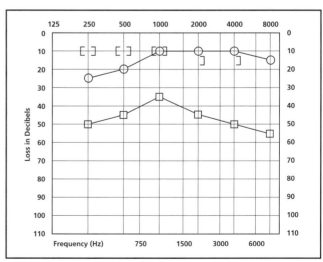

**Fig. 11-31
Perforated Tympanic Membrane**

11-8

Smaller perforations (right ear) affect only the low frequencies. As the hole increases in size (left ear), the conductive component spreads to all frequencies.

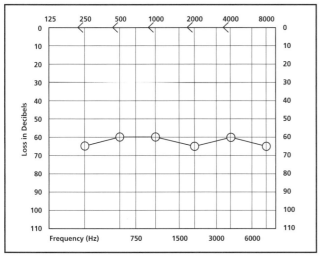

Fig. 11-32
Missing Drum and Ossicular Chain

A large hole in the eardrum and no ossicular chain produces a purely conductive loss, with up to 60 dB air-bone gap. The eardrum makes up about 20 dB, and the ossicular chain 40 dB.

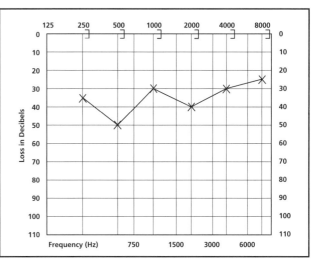

Fig. 11-33
Disarticulated Ossicular Chain

Disarticulation can occur between the malleus and the incus, or the incus and the stapes. The Tympanogram is Ad. With malleus involvement, a large conductive component with a 'V' notch occurs at 500 Hz. When the incudostapedial junction disarticulates, the 'V' conductive notch is at 2000 Hz.

DISTANCE LEARNING for Professionals in HEARING HEALTH SCIENCES

SPEECH TESTING

LESSON 12

The pure tone audiogram is only one indication of the extent of hearing impairment. It cannot be relied on entirely in the fitting of a hearing instrument for the following reasons. **Pure tone audiometry** measures the patient's responses to artificial tones - sounds that we rarely find in everyday life.

A **pure tone** is a sound that consists of only one frequency, produced by a tuning fork or an electronic instrument like an audiometer. Although pure tones sound artificial to us, they have the advantage of measuring the patient's capacity to hear a specific frequency without the involvement of other frequencies.

Pure tone measurements are **subjective.** Results depend entirely on the **patient's responses,** and motivation.

The audiogram gives you a picture of the patient's threshold responses at the faintest levels. Although you determine the pattern of hearing loss, you do not know about the hearing **levels where the patient normally listens.**

Most sounds we hear in our environment are a mixture of tones, or **complex sounds, like human speech,** and most musical instruments.

Speech audiometry is another indication of hearing function. Several formulas estimate the loss for speech from pure tone audiograms. These formulas serve as a check on the reliability of speech tests, but cannot substitute for them.

Normal Hearing The auditory area of man graph, (Figure 12-1), encompasses the normal range of usable hearing. Now you are looking at how normal ears process speech.

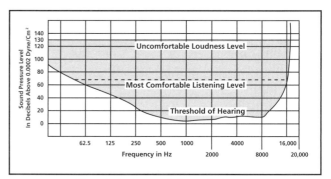

Fig. 12-1 Normal Speech Range

Speech Reception Threshold (SRT) The lower threshold of hearing differs at each frequency, just the same as the zero line on the audiogram.

Speech divides words into syllables, where a different accent is put on each syllable, i.e. DIE-hard, HARD-ly, HARD-en-er, HARD-ROCK. Local dialects or accents affect the pronunciation of syllables and words.

Speech Reception Threshold (SRT) is a point where spondaic words, or spondees, can be repeated 50% of the time. Spondaic words have two syllables, with equal stress or emphasis on each syllable, like baseball, hotdog, greyhound.

There is a level below SRT where you are aware someone is talking, but without enough frequencies represented to understand the words. **Speech Detection Threshold (SDT) or Speech Awareness Threshold (SAT),** about 8 - 10 dB lower than SRT, proves useful when testing anyone who does not speak English. SRT for normal ears is 20 dB SPL, (0 dB HL).

Uncomfortable Level (UCL): The upper boundary is the **Uncomfortable Level,** at about 130 dB SPL for normal ears. Sounds above this level cause discomfort, then pain. The range of usable hearing, between SRT and UCL, is the **Dynamic Range (DR), or Range of Comfortable**

Loudness. Calculate Dynamic Range by subtracting SRT from UCL, i.e. 130 - 20 = 110 dB dynamic range for normal ears. Usable hearing takes place within this dynamic range, or area of comfortable loudness. If the frequency and intensity of a sound are inside this area, we readily hear it. Any sound that falls below or outside this area, for example, 20,000 Hz, remains unheard.

Most Comfortable Level (MCL): The **Most Comfortable Level (MCL)** is approximately 65 dB SPL for normal ears, (45 dB HL).

Note that although MCL is 65 dB SPL, the range between threshold and MCL also differs at each frequency. At 250 Hz, MCL is 39.5 dB SPL **above threshold,** but it is 58 dB SPL above threshold at 1000 Hz, and 55.5 dB SPL above threshold at 4000 Hz. The low frequencies require less volume above threshold to become comfortable than the frequencies from 1000 Hz upward.

CONDUCTIVE LOSS

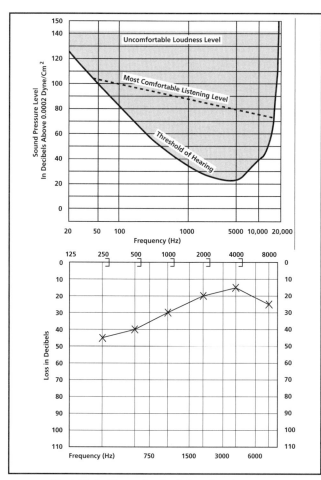

Fig. 12-2. Hypothetical Conductive Loss

A patient with a conductive loss has a blockage or occlusion that prevents the sound from reaching the inner ear, and the threshold of hearing elevates, greater in the lower frequencies. The patient needs sound louder to hear comfortably at MCL, and the UCL increases by the same amount. A conductive loss retains the wide dynamic range of normal ears, only every threshold elevates in the amount of the blockage.

SENSORINEURAL LOSS

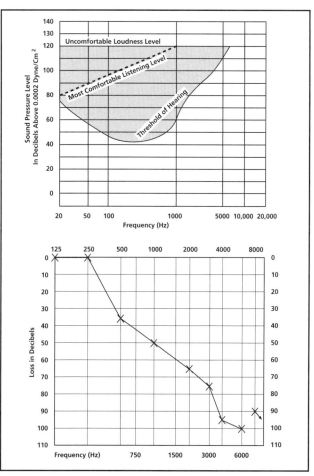

Fig. 12-3 Hypothetical Sensorineural Loss

The patient with a sensorineural loss usually has a greater loss in the higher frequencies than in the lows. MCL retains a relationship with the lower boundary, but now becomes slanted because of the altered shape of threshold. Also, as the threshold elevates, the UCL drops, forming a much narrower dynamic range. Now, MCL extends upward, past UCL, and into the area of discomfort. Obviously higher frequency sounds are NOT 'most comfortable,' they are intolerable. Yet, quieter sounds are not readily heard.

Some patients with sensorineural losses exhibit recruitment, an abnormally rapid increase in loudness as the intensity of a sound increases above threshold. The outer hair cells, vulnerable to ototoxic drugs and high noise levels, may cause this cochlear impairment.

COMPARISON of LOSSES

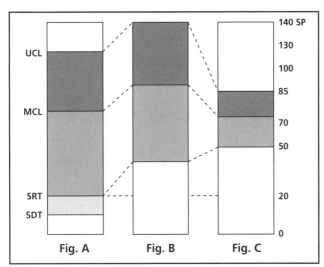

Fig. 12-4 Dynamic Range

The bar graph shows a comparison between normal, conductive, and sensorineural losses. **Fig. 12-4 A** shows a normal 110 dB Dynamic Range. **Fig. B,** the conductive loss, moves all of the dynamic range upward, often making it impossible to test true UCL. The sensorineural loss in **Fig. C** indicates how the dynamic range narrows to 35 dB or less.

A person with a dynamic range of 50 dB has no problem listening to recorded music, since most records produce about 35 dB range from the faintest to loudest sound. The volume is set at a comfortable level where the soft sounds can be heard and not bothered by the louder ones. This person has more difficulty with a live orchestra, with a dynamic range of 70 dB or greater. Sitting in the back, soft sounds would be missed, whereas moving closer, the person would be bothered by the loud sounds.

ANSI Standards: ANSI Standards for Speech testing are much simpler than for pure tones. **20 dB SPL = 0 dB HL.**

Now, lets look at the bar graphs again, converting to HL, and showing the limits of the audiometer.

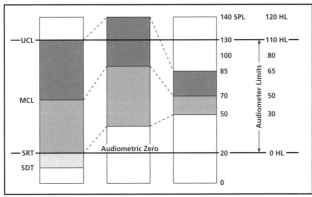

Fig. 12-5 Audiometer Limits

The Speech Awareness Threshold (SAT) or SDT would be hard to measure on normal ears because SRT is 0 dB HL. The limit of the audiometer may prevent the measurement of the uncomfortable level in a conductive hearing loss. Also notice that most comfortable level (MCL) is about half the dynamic range in both normal ears and those with hearing loss.

Speech Audiometry: Speech audiometry provides five types of information.

1. Speech Reception Threshold (SRT)
2. Most Comfortable Level (MCL)
3. Uncomfortable Level (UCL)
4. Dynamic Range (DR)
5. Speech Discrimination Score

Speech tests consist of presenting a series of words to the patient, asking the patient to repeat the words, and recording the responses repeated correctly.

MCL and UCL use continuous speech as a basis for determining these levels, although UCL can be tested at each frequency with a different stimulus.

Calculation is necessary to determine dynamic range: UCL - SRT = DR

Presentation. Speech audiometry uses monitored live voice, tapes or CD's, presented to the patient through the headset.

Monitored Live Voice. As the tester, you speak directly to the patient through the microphone, monitoring your voice with the VU Meter. The patient hears your voice through the headset, and responds according to your instructions. The attenuator dial controls the volume the patient hears, in dB HL.

Live voice testing requires a two-room suite, acoustically separated from the patient. Otherwise the patient hears your voice 'live', even though the voice via headphones is too quiet to hear, making results invalid.

A disadvantage of live voice testing is that you do not always speak the words the same way or with the same intensity. Different dialects or accents also affect the results.

Recorded Voice Testing Words are presented to the patient using tapes or CD's. The hearing level dial or attenuator controls the volume of the words, and the VU Meter displays the strength of presentation. There is a 1000 Hz calibration tone at the beginning of each tape or CD, allowing you to set the VU Meter at zero.

Testing requires only one room. Words are always at a consistent sound level, voice quality and enunciation. Your speech patterns do not affect the test results, making them repeatable from one tester to another.

Although live voice testing allows for the slower responses in the elderly, the 'pause' button on the tape recorder or CD works well when using recorded speech.

Recorded voice presentation is the method of choice, even with a two-room suite.

Speech Reception Threshold (SRT)

Purpose: You establish the lowest level that the patient can hear and understand speech.

SAT or SDT is a threshold where the patient is aware that speech is coming through the headset, but the level is too quiet to understand or repeat.

Instructions to the Patient "You are going to hear a person ask you to say a series of words, like 'greyhound' and 'schoolboy'. I'd like you to repeat each word you are asked to say. I'm going to turn the words quieter and quieter, until you can't repeat them any more. I want to find out how quietly you can hear speech. Don't be afraid to guess. Do you understand?"

Most people will not repeat the carrier phrase, 'Say the word', with these instructions. If they do repeat the carrier phrase more than twice, put the tape on 'pause'. switch to 'mike', and say "This may be easier if you only repeat the last word said. Is that OK with you?" Switch back to 'tape' and continue.

SRT equals PTA, plus or minus 5 dB. Normal range for SRT is 0 - 20 dB HL. Record the threshold, in dB HL, not the number of words correctly repeated.

Method: Begin testing at a level where the patient can hear and understand. To find threshold, decrease the volume of presentation in 10 dB steps, then bracket until you find the level the patient hears and correctly repeats spondaic words 50% of the time. A spondee has two syllables with equal stress on each syllable.

Masking SRT: Mask while testing the poorer ear whenever you used masking for pure tone air conduction testing. Use white noise or speech masking. Narrow band masking is not effective for speech tests. Effective masking is the SRT (or PTA, which should be the same) of the better ear, plus the cushion required for your audiometer.

Let your patient know that you are turning on the masking noise. Use the same instructions - "I'm going to put a noise into your good ear to keep it busy while I test your poorer ear. Pay no attention to the noise, just listen for and repeat the words."

If the patient has a dead ear, and does not respond, record CNT - could not test, or DNR - did not respond.

Most Comfortable Level (MCL): Most Comfortable Level (MCL) uses cold running speech as a stimulus. Cold running speech is an informative but non-emotional series of sentences, recorded at a constant level. Cold running speech carries a lot of **redundant information.** The patient hears and understands the subject without realizing that each individual word may not be clear. Many words could be left out of the sentence without losing meaning.

Because presentation of this speech is comfortable at any sensation level above SRT, a forced choice method determines a more accurate MCL.

Purpose: You want to determine the **best level** for the patient to hear and understand speech.

MCL gives important information both with regard to the patient, and to the fitting of a hearing instrument.

1. MCL represents about half of the dynamic range. Remember how the bar graphs illustrated MCL as approximately half-way up the dynamic range, although the DR changed for different types of losses.

2. The sensation level (SL) required to reach MCL is loaded with information. SL = MCL - SRT.

    a) Sensation level, times 2, should estimate the dynamic range.

    b) Sensation level can be a predicting factor in dis crimination scores.

    c) Sensation level verifies the type of audiogram, i.e., conductive losses have a greater SL than sensorineural losses.

Instructions to the Patient: "Now you are going to hear continuous speech. You do not have to repeat any of the words. I want to find the most comfortable level for you to listen. I will increase the volume slowly, so you can listen at different levels. You can help me by pointing your finger up if you want it louder, or down when you want it quieter. Please let me know when we find the volume you prefer. Do you understand?"

Forced Choice Method. Always advance the attenuator dial to a point a little above where the patient reports speech as most comfortable. While really listening quietly, realization may come to the patient that speech can be louder and perhaps more comfortable. Continue to increase slowly in 5 dB steps until the patient decides speech was better lower, then return to that level.

Masking MCL: Whenever masking was used for air conduction tests, masking is required for MCL. Effective masking is the MCL of the good ear, plus your cushion, or 70 dB SPL, whichever is less. As normal conversational speech is about 65 dB SPL, this masking level covers normal conversational speech.

Uncomfortable Level (UCL): UCL is **not** the threshold of pain; it is a level where speech becomes uncomfortably loud.

For normal ears, the **threshold of pain** is about 130 - 140 dB SPL or 110 - 120 dB HL. The **threshold of tickle** or **threshold of feeling** is 120 - 130 dB SPL or 100 - 110 dB HL. These levels are 20 - 30 dB above where sound becomes uncomfortably loud.

Uncomfortable level (UCL) for our purposes goes by many names:

LDL - loudness discomfort level,

TD - threshold of discomfort,

Purpose: To find the upper limit of the dynamic range, a point where no further amplification will be permitted in a hearing instrument or accepted by the patient.

Instructions to the Patient: You are not looking for the level 5 dB above MCL, where the patient says 'That's too loud." Your instructions to the patient are critical to this measurement.

"Now I want to find a level where sound starts to bother you, not where it is a little bit too loud. I want you to be able to hear a telephone ring, or a fire alarm, but I don't want you to hold your ears in pain. Please raise your hand, or say 'stop' whenever the sound starts to bother you."

Masking UCL: Use the masking level required for MCL whenever you have to mask air conduction thresholds.

Converting Speech Levels to SPL: SRT, MCL and UCL all convert to SPL by adding 20 dB. (ANSI Standards). SL needs no conversion, as this level relates to the threshold of the patient, not HL or SPL. Binaural MCL is usually 5 dB less than monaural MCL. Both SRT and UCL change as well.

SRT lowers binaurally because of binaural summation. UCL can lower, or become more comfortable because the sound appears to move out and away from the ear. The definition of UCL is where the patient is bothered by sound, not the threshold of pain. Always check your UCL's in the final fitting and verification of the hearing instrument.

The speech tests you have learned so far are possible to do on anyone, regardless of whether they speak English or not. Although SRT requires the patient to repeat spondee words, SAT or SDT does not require anything but an awareness of speech being present. The addition of 8 - 10 dB to a SDT score estimates SRT nicely.

Cold running speech can be comfortable or uncomfortable in any language, regardless of whether it is understood. It is always possible to calculate dynamic range. Instructions to the patient can be by hand signals. SAT requires only that you hold your thumb and finger close together. MCL reads 'OK' by forming a circle with your thumb and finger and the rest of the fingers extended. For louder - point up, quieter - point down. UCL needs no explanation if you watch closely for facial expression. If MCL is a problem, divide the dynamic range by two for an estimate.

When testing an English speaking patient, the spondaic words are easy to understand at very quiet levels. Cold running speech has so much redundancy that it is easy to follow.

Each of these tests help you to verify the accuracy of your audiogram:

SRT verifies your pure tone average.

SL to MCL often exceeds 40 dB with normal thresholds, or conductive losses.

Mixed losses choose a 30 - 40 dB SL unless only one or two frequencies are involved, then they respond as a sensorineural loss. Large conductive components respond more like conductive losses.

Sensorineural losses have a narrower dynamic range, usually picking 30 dB SL or less. When a patient chooses less than 30 dB, consider this choice to be a **red flag.** His UCL is not far away.

Are each of your tests supporting the audiogram, type of loss, case history information, tympanograms and visual inspection?

Speech Discrimination: Speech discrimination tests use single syllable word lists, chosen so they approximate a sample of speech sounds occurring in an ordinary conversation. These words have no redundancy, and are hard to discriminate unless they are loud enough.

As human speech and most musical instruments are complex sounds, we need to understand the factors involved in hearing and discriminating complex sounds.

Timbre: The timbre or tonal quality of a complex sound depends on:

1. the number of frequencies in the complex sound,

2. the relative strength of each of these frequencies, and

3. the resonance of the chamber surrounding the sound.

The timbre or tonal quality is what makes a violin sound different from a flute, even though they both produce the same frequency and intensity. The timbre of sounds produced in these instruments also involves the resonance of the cavities of the flute and violin.

Fundamental Frequency: In a complex tone, the lowest frequency, being the loudest, predominates. The frequency that predominates is the **fundamental frequency.** The weaker, higher frequency components are **overtones.** Overtones in exact multiples of the fundamental frequency are **harmonics.**

For example, a complex tone with a fundamental frequency of 200 Hz has harmonics at 400 Hz, 600 Hz, 800 Hz, etc.

A clarinet has a strong fundamental frequency, a weak, barely present second harmonic, a third harmonic almost as strong as the fundamental, and a nearly absent fourth harmonic. The combination and relative strength of harmonics give the clarinet its unique timbre or tonal quality.

In contrast, the violin fundamental tone is strong, the second harmonic almost as strong, the third harmonic weak, and the fourth stronger than the third. The violin's timbre has different harmonics, and cannot sound like a clarinet.

Speech Sounds: Each speech sound, or **phoneme,** is composed of several frequencies of varying intensities. For example, we recognize the different vowel sounds because of the variations in timbre. The fundamental frequency can change, depending on whether we are speaking or singing.

Fourier Spectral Analysis gives us a way to show energy at different frequencies in complex sounds. A line spectrum graphically represents the relative strengths of harmonics in a complex sound.

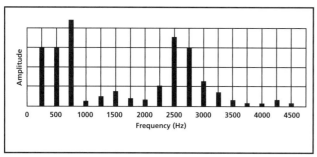

Fig. 13-1 Line Spectrum

The line spectrum shows the different frequencies and their intensities for the vowel sound 'a,' as in the word 'tape'. Note the concentration of energy around 250 - 750 Hz, and also 2500 - 2750 Hz. These concentrations of energy are **formants.**

Formants: A formant is a range of frequencies in the spectrum of a sound where certain harmonics are relatively loud. Formants give complex sounds their distinctive characteristics, enabling us to differentiate one musical instrument from another, or one vowel from another.

The most important energy for recognizing speech sounds are the second and third formants. These spectral energy peaks, produced by the resonance of the vocal tract of the speaker, contain relatively weak high frequency components of speech above 1000 Hz.

Formant transitions are the movement of these energy peaks to other frequency regions as the shape of the speakers' vocal tract changes for another phoneme.

Most hearing losses affect recognition of these mid and high frequency phonemes, and without these critical clues, greatly reduce the ability to discriminate speech.

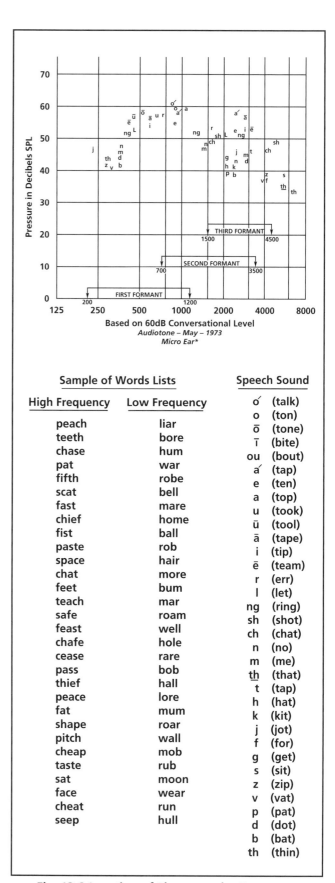

Fig. 13-2 Location of Phonemes by Frequency

When plotting the frequency regions and relative volume of speech sounds on a chart, some sounds have more than one frequency component, appearing in both low and high areas on the chart. The most powerful sounds are 'aw' (o´) as in 'talk', 'uh' (o) as in 'ton', 'oh' (ō) as in 'tone', 'ah' (a´) as in 'tap', 'a' (ā) as in 'tape', 'oo' (ū) as in 'tool', and 'r'. The weakest sounds, 'z, s, v, f', and 'th' as in 'thin' - the weakest of all speech sounds, only appear in the high frequencies. The '<u>th</u>' as in 'that' also has a low frequency component.

Low frequency phonemes appear louder than those in the higher frequencies. You can say an 'oh' very loudly, but have difficulty getting any volume with a 'p' or 't' in 'put'. Because background noise has most of the energy in the low frequencies, it easily masks out the weaker high frequency phonemes. People with cochlear hearing loss have greater difficulty understanding speech in noisy backgrounds than those with normal hearing or conductive hearing loss. Most of the energy in low frequencies of background noise masks out the weaker high frequency components.

The upward spread of masking occurs whenever a low frequency sound masks out a higher frequency sound. The higher frequencies in speech are always more important for providing intelligibility than the lower frequencies.

If a low frequency phoneme is disproportionately louder than a higher frequency phoneme, as in a high frequency hearing loss, then the louder, lower frequency phonemes also mask out the weaker, higher frequency sounds.

Backward masking results when a louder sound occurs immediately after a softer sound, causing the softer sound to be inaudible, even though it occurred first.

Forward masking occurs when one sound follows another closely in time and the first sound reduces the sensitivity of recently stimulated cells.

When fitting a hearing instrument, problems arise when some first formants of speech are over-amplified, drowning out the higher frequency speech formants, and causing speech to mask itself. Some or all of these masking situations occur unless amplified speech is in the proper intensities.

Intensity vs Discrimination

Once speech is loud enough to hear, does the volume or intensity of the speech have any effect on discrimination?

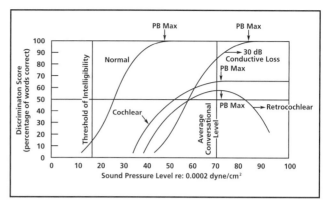

Fig. 13-3 Performance-intensity functions for normal ear, conductive loss, cochlear site of lesion, and retrocochlear site of lesion.

Note the vertical line at 70 dB SPL, average conversational level. Normal hearing is 100% at this level. A person with a 30 dB conductive loss gets 85% of the words, a cochlear loss hears just over 60% of the words, and a retrocochlear loss discriminates about 55% of the words. This chart gives us data on what to expect on an unaided discrimination test with each type of hearing loss.

The sensation level to MCL acts as a predictor of discrimination scores. Instructions in most text books suggest a 40 dB SL, a 30 dB SL, or MCL. Hopefully, your patient will wear the hearing instrument at MCL. The information most helpful in the fitting involves the discrimination scores at MCL. If you want to find out if a patient has a cochlear or retrocochlear loss, a second discrimination test at a higher level supplies this information. This second score, usually at 90 dB, tests **Pb Roll-over,** where retrocochlear losses lose their already poor ability to discriminate.

Using monitored live voice is acceptable, although recorded words are the method of choice.

Instructions to the Patient: "You are going to hear a series of words. Please repeat each of the words you are asked to say. If you have difficulty understanding the words, it helps me if you guess. I have a better idea what part of the word was difficult for you. If the volume is not comfortable for you, or you would like the words louder or quieter, please let me know. Do you understand?"

Some patients find cold running speech comfortable, but, when asked to discriminate words, ask for more volume. When the patient asks you to adjust the volume, mark the new level down, and begin 25 words at the new volume.

Scoring the Test: Allow 2% for each of the words correctly repeated on a 50 word list. If you use only 25 words, each word is 4%. Record each incorrect answer. Any response other than the word presented, for example, changing a singular to a plural, or vice versa, is an error, and marked wrong. Do not consider accents to be valid errors. If, during the case history, the patient says 'dis' and 'dat' for 'this' and 'that', do not expect the patient to say 'there' correctly.

Masking: Use masking levels for MCL whenever you required masking in air conduction tests. Indicate the type and amount used on the audiogram.

Binaural Testing: Sometimes patients with fairly similar audiograms and other speech test results will differ greatly in discrimination scores between ears. If your audiometer has two intensity dials, you have the capability of testing a binaural discrimination. You want to determine if the discrimination of the poorer ear helps or confuses the better ear when listening with both ears together at binaural MCL. If the discrimination score drops, the patient usually has difficulty adjusting to a hearing instrument in both ears.

Patients with no differences between ears can also have improved binaural scores. The Speech Discrimination score becomes an important criterion for deciding which ear to fit, or if a binaural fitting is superior to either ear, alone.

Do not assume that an ear with better air conduction thresholds, or better SRT's have better discrimination. The patient may be able to hear the words without being able to understand them.

Fundamental Frequency (ff) - lowest frequency in a complex sound displaying the most energy.

Octave - Doubling of a frequency.

Example: 125 Hz x 2 = 250 Hz (an octave)

250 Hz x 2 = 500 Hz (an octave)

Harmonic - Simple Integral Multiple of a frequency. The adding of the frequency to itself.

Example: 125 Hz + 125 Hz = 250 Hz (an harmonic)

250 Hz + 125 Hz = 375 Hz (an harmonic)

375 Hz + 125 Hz = 500 Hz (an harmonic)

Overtone - Any frequency found above the fundamental frequency (ff).

Example: 125 Hz ff

Octave	Harmonics	Overtones
		130 Hz
		150 Hz
		240 Hz
250 Hz	250 Hz	250 Hz
		260 Hz
		370 Hz
	375 Hz	375 Hz
500 Hz	500 Hz	500 Hz
	625 Hz	625 Hz
		700 Hz
	750 Hz	750 Hz
	875 Hz	875 Hz
		890 Hz
1000 Hz	1000 Hz	1000 Hz

All frequencies above the fundamental frequency are overtones. Only specific frequencies may be octaves and/or harmonics.

Tympanometry is the first test procedure in the battery of evaluative methods and is part of the group known as Otoimmitance Measurements. It follows a thorough history and otoscopy (either video or manual). It is the most commonly used of these methods, having found great utility in screening, as part of the larger battery of clinical procedures, and, as an electrophysiologic measure of external and middle ear function. Tympanometry identifies a measure of the dynamic compliance of the tympanic membrane (TM) and reflects the algebraic sum of the factors influencing middle ear performance.

When used in the "screening" of patients (for whatever reason) it addresses the question: "Should this patient be referred for medical follow-up?" As such, in combination with the thorough history, it is a quick and powerful tool in the hands of the adept professional. When the full group of procedures within this paradigm is utilized, it contributes, significantly to identification of otopathology in a number of anatomic locations.

PROCEDURE:

A closed chamber is created with the TM at the medial end, and a metal probe [covered with a soft plastic tip called the "probe tip'] at the other. The walls of the closed chamber are skin over either bone or cartilage. Sound is introduced into the chamber through the probe tip and then measured as the TM is manipulated through a prescribed range of motions. Positive and negative water pressure levels are exerted against the TM to attempt to elicit movement through this range. By convention, that range is from + 200mm H2O - through 0 mm H20 to -200mm H20. Although this range can be extended more negatively, - 200 mm H2O is sufficient for the meeting of referral criterion.

When the maximum positive pressure (+200 mm H20) is introduced into the chamber (or cavity) and exerted against the TM, it causes it to be moved the maximum distance from the probe tip. It becomes stiffened by the combination of resistance and reactance, and reflects acoustic energy introduced to it back out toward the probe. Since energy transfer through the TM is limited, the sound is described as "quiet" or "soft".

When there is neither positive nor negative pressure (0 mm H20) exerted, the TM is free to move, unfettered, if you will. If the position of the TM is "normal" this neutral pressure status permits the maximum passage of acoustic energy through. At that point, therefore the sound is "loudest". The "peak" reflects the "point of maximum compliance" of the membrane.

This point of maximum compliance is always achieved when the pressure exerted in the chamber matches the pressure level in the middle ear. It is at this point that the sound is perceived as being "loudest. It is from this location (at which the curve of the tympanogram changes direction) that we are able to infer the status of middle ear pressure.

When the maximum negative pressure (- 200 mm H20) is exerted the TM is being "pulled" out into the canal and again, becomes stiffened by the combination of the shape and resistance of the TM itself. It also reflects acoustic energy introduced to it back out toward the probe. There the sound is (once again) "quiet".

The physics of this involve an understanding of how the TM moves (or does not) through a specific range of motion. It is also important to comprehend the transmittal of energy from acoustic (sound), through mechanical (after the interface of the TM) in the ossicular chain, and then, through the additional interface of the oval window membrane, into hydraulic energy in cochlea in the inner ear.

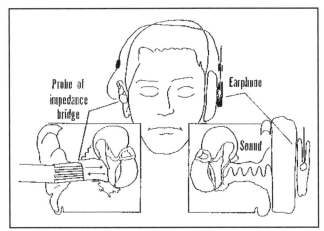

Fig. 14-1

The physical mechanism for it is based upon a measurement of the sound pressure level within the ear canal (and elicited changes therein). (Fig. 14-1)

Tympanometry is used, almost without exception, in the dispensing practice of audiologists and dispensers. In my opinion, it belongs in every dispensing office as a proper tool for the identification of otopathology. It provides more, and better quality information about the necessity for referral, faster than any other single procedure in the armamentarium of the practitioner.

THE PROCEDURE

The procedure is quite simple. After a thorough history in which past ear surgery is explored, an otoscopic examination is conducted. (Note: NEVER put an otoimmittance probe {or probe tip} into an ear without first, looking into that ear). Following the inspection, a soft malleable tip which covers the metallic end of the "probe" is selected, slightly larger than the external canal diameter, to form an hermetic "seal" at the canal opening. Of all of the parts of the battery of otoimmitance measurements, this (correct initial selection of a probe "tip") seems to be the most confusing. We find it easier to do if the decision is made based upon the perception of the distended diameter of the canal. That perception springs from observation of the shape of the canal when the posterior superior margin of the pinna is grasped and stretched (slightly) up, and to the rear (in adults), and "down" by pulling on the lobe - (slightly) in children five or younger.

Once a seal is obtained, the generation of the tympanogram is rapid. If an automatic instrument is used, the seal itself initiates the process by which air pressure is varied across a range from +200 mmH2O to -200 (or 400) mmH2O. The sound pressure level in the cavity formed by the TM (at the medial end) and the probe tip (at the lateral end) will vary as the TM is moved through the range of pressures. The tympanogram is a graph of that sound pressure level variation across those pressures. In fact, otoacoustic immitance information is based solely upon measurements of the sound pressure level within that cavity. (Fig. 14-2)

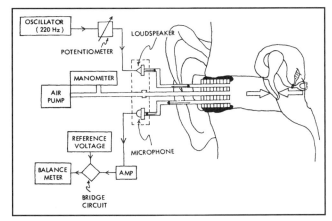

Fig. 14-2 - Electroacoustic immittance meter. Note Probe sealed into external auditory meatus with three holes for (a) 220-Hz probe tone from oscillator; (b) air pressure system from air pump and manometer; and (c) pick-up microphone to compare sound pressure level in the cavity between the eardrum and probe tip with the reference voltage of impedance bridge. (Reprinted with permission from J. Jerger: Archives of Otolaryngology 92: 311-324, 1970.)

Once the tympanogram is generated, comparison of the elicited graph with the normative data can be made. This comparison, along with accompanying information about the presence or absence of middle ear muscle reflexes, permits statements to be made about the auditory system as both a mechanical system and in regard to its neurological competence. It is important, at this point, to make some observations.

1) Tympanometry is not a hearing test. It is possible for a dead ear to produce a normal tympanogram.

2) Middle ear muscles (i.e., the stapedial reflex), in general, require acoustic stimulation (hearing) for activation of that activity, even under the most "normal" of middle ear conditions.

3) The patient can be awake or asleep, and the results will be the same.

COMPARATIVE INTERPRETATION

The comparison of a measured tympanogram with normative patterns, in combination with middle ear muscle reflex data, permit a significant amount of information to be inferred (NOTE: the information is always inferential).

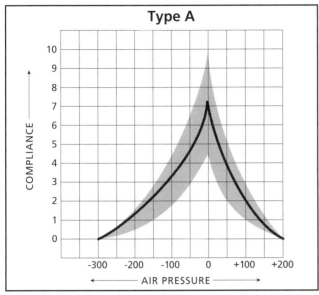

Fig. 14-3

Type A ("Normal") tympanograms (Fig. 14-3) require an intact TM. They require the presence of air in the middle ear space, and therefore, function of the eustachean tube that is within the range of normal limits. They require that bones and muscles, ligaments and tendons of the middle ear be present, intact and functioning, as well. In general the range of static compliance runs from about 0.4cc to roughly 1.6cc of equivalent volume (allowing for individual variation).

Type As ("Shallow A") tympanograms (Fig. 14-4) require all of the above except that the transfer of energy through the system is somewhat impeded by an increased "stiffness". Although there is still an identifiable peak to the tympanogram shape, the static compliance measurement is markedly reduced ranging up to approximately 0.4cc (of equivalent volume).

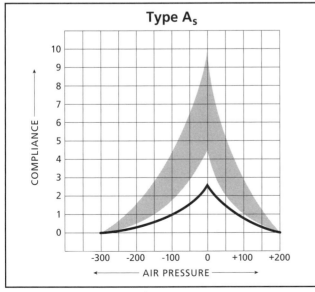

Fig. 14-4

Ossicular fixation (stapedial, incudal or malleolar fixation) and/ or tympanosclerosis (calcium deposits on the surface of the TM), create increased stiffness in the movement of the system. Since the ossicular chain is a Class II lever - ATTACHED at it's lateral margin to the medial surface of the tympanic membrane, ANYTHING which modifies the efficiency of the transfer of energy through the system changes the impedance matching characteristics of the middle ear. We describe such a loss of efficiency as a "Conductive Hearing problem (Loss)". Other possible causes could be scar tissue or thickened epithelial tissue on the lateral margin of the TM.

Type Ad ("Deep A") tympanograms (Fig. 14-5) also require an intact TM as well as normal eustachean tube function. However, resistance to the flow of energy is smaller-than-normal through the system. The location and mobility of the tympanic membrane is dependent upon a complex algebraic summation of the vector forces of mass, resistance and reactance. Static compliance measures identified in these cases fall above 1.6 cc of equivalent volume and again, represent an impedance matching transformer in which the efficiency has been reduced.

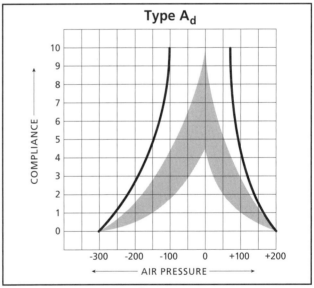

Fig. 14-5

The two most common, causative, factors of this pattern are:

1) Ossicular discontinuity, or an incomplete "chain" causing "flaccid" movement of the membrane.

   and/or

2) A Monomeric membrane, in which a recovering perforation produces a weak spot when the epithelial (or outer) layer grows back.

In this instance, as well, we infer - from the measured sound pressure level in the cavity between the medial end of the probe tip and the lateral layer of the TM -

conditions existent "behind" that membrane. We are assisted in this regard by the fact that the monomer is visible (upon careful otoscopic examination).

It is reluctantly noted, that this pattern of tympanogram is also commonly seen in those cases of "abuse" which have included a blow to the ear. Typically, in such cases, the patient is seen AFTER the actual facial "bruising" has faded, but (perhaps) still in time for the lividity marks to remain in the post-auricular hairline.

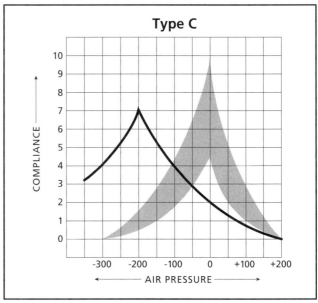

Fig. 14-7

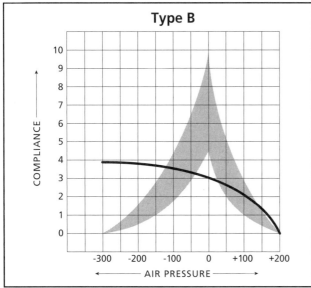

Fig. 14-6

Type B tympanograms (Fig. 14-6) can occur for a number of reasons. These include, but are not limited to: obstruction in the canal, perforation of the TM, middle ear fluid (including serous or adhesive fluid, suppurative [as a result of an acute infection] or blood/lymph secondary to traumatic injury), or atelectasis (over-retraction) of the TM. In addition, misapplication of the probe tip can also produce a false-positive Type B pattern.

Type C tympanograms (Fig. 14-7) also require all of the above (intact membrane, etc.) except there is a substantial negative pressure in the middle ear space, usually referred to as a retracted tympanic membrane. Subjective symptoms include pressure, fullness, "hollowness", and a decrease in hearing.

Type C is usually identified in an ear that is "in transition". When the middle ear muscle reflexes are present in this condition, it may be considered to be "recovering". On the other hand, when these reflexes are absent, the ear may be said to be "getting worse". In a short period of time (perhaps - by tomorrow,) it will become a Type B. In either a Type B or a Type C (without middle ear muscle reflexes), medical referral is the indicated procedure.

There is value in the practice of interpreting the information generated with your own (specific) equipment. We use this equipment for our screening work in schools, nursing homes, the hospital and in the hearing aid practice. Our clinical equipment enables the more explicit and differential evaluation of cochlear, VIIIth nerve and low auditory brainstem auditory pathway locations which permits inferential understanding of the anatomy and physiology of the system. Tympanometry is the quickest and most efficient means of identifying those cases which need to be referred for medical treatment. This is especially true of middle ear pathology of any kind.

There is a tendency to forget (or ignore) that population who are incapable (or unwilling) to provide reliable and consistent behavioral responses. This group (which include both the very young and the very old, as well as those with head injury, trauma, dementia, and others) have serious need for effective and accurate evaluation. Moreover, middle ear muscle reflex measurements are also often the first indicant of those cases which later turn out to involve the VIIIth Cranial Nerve and/or the low portion of the auditory brainstem pathways. They are also often the first indicators of demyelenating disease.

Tympanometric shape is also a factor in matrix modification when ordering and fitting the hearing aid. When fitting in-the-ear, in-the-canal and deep insertion hearing aids, control of output is so critical that 2 - 3dB (at a frequency at which the ear is recruiting) may represent the difference between success or failure. When controlling the output of an hearing instrument, we look at the shape of tympanogram, translating the height of the tympanogram (and volume of it's static compliance) into a means of "fine tuning" the instrument.

If there is a tympanogram of Type A which has a high peak (not uncommon in highly mobile tympanic membranes) we request a measured reduction in the output of the instrument of about 2 - 3 dB. This is because the transfer of energy through the middle ear mechanism is highly efficient, and (therefore) more energy passes through. On the other hand, when there is a TM through which energy passes less efficiently than might be normal (as in the Type As, or A "shallow"), we request a small addition in the capacity for output. This allows us to be able to compensate for the additional "stiffness" of the system.

At the outset of this section we made reference to the fact that tympanometry was simply the first of the battery of procedures referred to as otoimmitance measures.

Acoustic Middle Ear Muscle Reflex Threshold Measurements, Non-Acoustic Middle Ear Muscle Reflex identification, Acoustic Middle Ear Muscle Reflex Decay Measurements, Eustachean Tube Function tests, Acoustic Middle Ear Muscle Reflex Latency tests, and even a version of a test for Perilymph Fistula, have a place within the capability of some versions of the equipment.

In addition, the use of the acoustic middle ear muscle reflex for the differential control of volume in the fitting of the hearing instrument and/or the differential height of the tympanogram for the "fine tuning" of output (when taken in combination with the experience of the patient with such devices) can be done, as well (when needed) as a predictive technique (the Sensitivity Prediction from the Acoustic Reflex [SPAR]) for identification of the degree and slope of loss (through the speech frequencies) in patients who are physically (or cognitively) unable to respond.

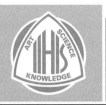
TEST INSTRUCTIONS

After you have finished reading this lesson, carefully study the selections from the **Required Reading.**

Then, look over the lesson once more to impress the important points on your memory.

When you are sure you know the lesson thoroughly, use the answer sheet in the back of the manual that corresponds to this lesson.

IMPORTANT: Place your student number on the answer sheets. Your student number appears on the inside front cover of the manual. **It must appear on your answer sheets in order for you to get credit for completion of the lesson.**

Once the answer sheet is completed, tear it out and mail to: International Institute for Hearing Instruments Studies
16880 Middlebelt Road, Suite 4, Livonia, MI 48154-3367

REQUIRED READING FOR THIS LESSON

Pages 73-105 – **Hearing Instrument Science and Fitting Practices (Second Edition)**

Pages 9-12 – **Masking (Third Edition)**

Pages 48-49 – **Introduction to the Auditory System**

TEST QUESTIONS

1. **A dial on the audiometer to control the decibels of output is called:**
    a. a frequency dial
    b. a hearing level dial
    c. an attenuator dial
    d. b & c above

2. **Audiometric zero for pure tones is higher than the standard reference level by about:**
    a. 35 dB
    b. 20 dB
    c. 10 dB
    d. differs at each frequency

3. **ANSI letters stand for:**
    a. Amplitude Narrowing in Short Increments
    b. Alternate Non Sensitive Intensities
    c. American National Safety Institute
    d. American National Standards Institute

4. **The audiometer is designed so that zero on the attenuator dial:**
   a. corresponds to the same sound pressure level at each audiometer frequency
   b. represents the level of normal hearing for that frequency
   c. represents where the best ear can hear
   d. you hear no sound when the dial is at 0

5. **By air conduction, sound energy changes forms in which of the following manners:**
   a. acoustic energy, mechanical energy, chemical energy, electrical energy to hydraulic energy
   b. mechanical energy, acoustic energy, chemical energy, hydraulic energy to electrical energy
   c. acoustic energy, mechanical energy, hydraulic energy, electrical energy to chemical energy
   d. electrical energy, mechanical energy, acoustic energy, hydraulic energy to chemical energy

6. **The normal ear responds to a range of frequencies from:**
   a. 15-50,000 Hz
   b. 20-20,000 Hz
   c. 20-30,000 Hz
   d. 30-30,000 Hz

7. **Sound waves, during bone conduction, transmit from the:**
   a. skull to the cochlea
   b. ossicles to the cochlea
   c. pinna to the ossicles
   d. skull to the eighth nerve

8. **Which of the following describes a Phon?**
   a. A unit of measurement when comparing the loudness of one frequency to another frequency
   b. A unit of measurement to determine the just noticeable difference (JND)
   c. A unit to measure loudness
   d. A unit of measurement for comparing the threshold of audibility with the threshold of comfort

9. **Routine hearing testing should be performed:**
   a. in an anechoic chamber
   b. in the home environment
   c. in a sound controlled environment
   d. in a room with a sound meter

10. **Audiometric zero is:**
    a. 0 dB Hearing Level
    b. 0 dB HL
    c. the level where normal ears can hear at every frequency
    d. all of the above

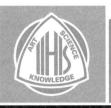
TEST INSTRUCTIONS

After you have finished reading this lesson, carefully study the selections from the **Required Reading.**

Then, look over the lesson once more to impress the important points on your memory.

When you are sure you know the lesson thoroughly, use the answer sheet in the back of the manual that corresponds to this lesson.

IMPORTANT: Place your student number on the answer sheets. Your student number appears on the inside front cover of the manual. **It must appear on your answer sheets in order for you to get credit for completion of the lesson.**

Once the answer sheet is completed, tear it out and mail to: International Institute for Hearing Instruments Studies
16880 Middlebelt Road, Suite 4, Livonia, MI 48154-3367

REQUIRED READING FOR THIS LESSON

Pages 100-127 – **Hearing Instrument Science and Fitting Practices (Second Edition)**

Pages 8-12 – **Masking (Third Edition)**

Pages 51-56 – **Introduction to the Auditory System**

TEST QUESTIONS

1. **In Pure Tone testing, threshold means:**
   a. the lowest intensity the client hears 50% of the time
   b. the sound has a loudness of zero dB in a 2 cc coupler
   c. the point at which the client reports the sound as most comfortable
   d. 0 dB HL

2. **What is the meaning of 40 dB threshold re: audiometric zero, at 500 Hz?**
   a. subject could not hear a 500 Hz tone at 40 dB
   b. subject could barely hear a 500 Hz tone at 40 dB about 50% of the time
   c. subject could hear a 500 Hz tone very well at 40 dB, and 5 dB lower
   d. subject could hear a 500 Hz tone with the hearing dial set at zero

3. **The problems produced by excessive ambient noise are:**
   a. greater for the lower frequencies than the higher frequencies
   b. greater for the higher frequencies than the lower frequencies
   c. affecting both high and low frequencies equally
   d. not a problem because a headset covers the ears

4. **Before testing is done:**
   a. the client's ears should be carefully examined using an otoscope
   b. you should carefully remove any impacted cerumen, if the client so requests
   c. you should hand the earphones to the client so that he can put them on in a comfortable manner
   d. none of the above

5. **The descending technique in pure tone audiometry is preferred because it:**
   a. is easier to hear when a sound stops than when it begins
   b. is the easier for the operator to explain to the client
   c. can prevent 'hearing fatigue'
   d. all of the above

6. **Begin testing with the 1000 Hz tone because it:**
   a. is the center frequency of those most important to understanding speech
   b. has good test re-test reliability
   c. provides the opportunity for the client to become accustomed to the procedure
   d. all of the above

7. **The symbols used in the audiogram for air conduction are:**
   a. uniform for the United States only
   b. uniform for Europe only
   c. uniform worldwide
   d. a circle for the left, and x for the right

8. **Individuals with a noise induced hearing impairment can have a 'V' notch at which frequency?**
   a. 3000 Hz
   b. 4000 Hz
   c. 6000 Hz
   d. any of the above

9. **The loss of acoustic energy as it travels from the test ear to the non-test ear is a definition of:**
   a. tonal deficiency effect
   b. interaural attenuation
   c. occlusion effect
   d. auditory fatigue

10. **To begin testing for air or bone conduction thresholds, tests should begin at which frequency?**
    a. 1000 Hz
    b. 2000 Hz
    c. 500 Hz
    d. 250 Hz

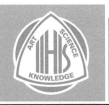

DISTANCE LEARNING for PROFESSIONALS in HEARING HEALTH SCIENCES

Lesson 9 — Pure Tone Bone Conduction Tests

TEST INSTRUCTIONS

After you have finished reading this lesson, carefully study the selections from the **Required Reading.**

Then, look over the lesson once more to impress the important points on your memory.

When you are sure you know the lesson thoroughly, use the answer sheet in the back of the manual that corresponds to this lesson.

IMPORTANT: Place your student number on the answer sheets. Your student number appears on the inside front cover of the manual. **It must appear on your answer sheets in order for you to get credit for completion of the lesson.**

Once the answer sheet is completed, tear it out and mail to: International Institute for Hearing Instruments Studies
16880 Middlebelt Road, Suite 4, Livonia, MI 48154-3367

REQUIRED READING FOR THIS LESSON

Pages 114-128
Hearing Instrument Science and Fitting Practices (Second Edition)
Pages 57-60 and 74-75 – **Introduction to the Auditory System**

TEST QUESTIONS

1. **If the outer and middle ear parts are normal:**
   a. air thresholds will equal the bone thresholds
   b. air thresholds will be better than bone thresholds
   c. air thresholds will be worse than bone thresholds
   d. you cannot measure bone thresholds

2. **In bone conduction testing, the receiver should be:**
   a. placed so that it is in contact with the pinna as well as the mastoid
   b. held in place by the person being tested
   c. placed at the most sensitive spot on the mastoid of the test ear
   d. held in place by a headband that exerts exactly one pound of pressure

3. **Sounds from the bone conduction receiver may stimulate the non-test ear at:**
   a. 10 dB or less
   b. 20 dB - 30 dB
   c. 30 dB - 40 dB
   d. 40 dB or more

4. **A source of information that helps to identify which ear is responding to bone conduction stimuli is:**
   a. tympanometry
   b. acoustic reflex testing
   c. bone conduction with masking
   d. all of the above

5. **Bone conduction testing directly stimulates:**
   a. the middle ear
   b. semi-circular canals
   c. the cochlea
   d. the pinna

6. **Most conductive losses:**
   a. are medically correctable
   b. display a breakdown or obstruction in the middle ear
   c. display good discrimination
   d. all of the above

7. **Ambient noise in the environment during bone conduction testing will:**
   a. affect the test results in the lower frequencies
   b. affect the test results in the mid frequencies
   c. affect the test results in the high frequencies
   d. all of the above

8. **During the testing process, it is best to test bone conduction:**
   a. before air conduction testing
   b. after air conduction testing
   c. after the case history
   d. after impedance audiometry

9. **A conductive loss may be caused by:**
   a. perforations of the tympanic membrane
   b. immobile middle ear ossicles
   c. otitis media
   d. all of the above

10. **Bone conduction thresholds worse than air conduction thresholds may be caused by:**
    a. poor placement of the vibrator
    b. a skull fracture
    c. thickness of the skull
    d. all of the above

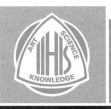

TEST INSTRUCTIONS

After you have finished reading this lesson, carefully study the selections from the **Required Reading.**

Then, look over the lesson once more to impress the important points on your memory.

When you are sure you know the lesson thoroughly, use the answer sheet in the back of the manual that corresponds to this lesson.

IMPORTANT: Place your student number on the answer sheets. Your student number appears on the inside front cover of the manual. **It must appear on your answer sheets in order for you to get credit for completion of the lesson.**

Once the answer sheet is completed, tear it out and mail to: International Institute for Hearing Instruments Studies
16880 Middlebelt Road, Suite 4, Livonia, MI 48154-3367

REQUIRED READING FOR THIS LESSON
Pages 5-25, 42-47
Masking (Third Edition)
Pages 3-9, 25-26, 46-48, 92 & 93
Hearing Instrument Science and Fitting Practices (Second Edition)

TEST QUESTIONS

1. **Sound being presented to one ear and then routed to the opposite ear is known as:**
   a. cross hearing
   b. shadow hearing
   c. transcranial hearing
   d. all of the above

2. **When the better ear 'answers' for the poorer ear what occurs?**
   a. shadow curve
   b. central hearing
   c. overmasking
   d. interaural attenuation

3. **Which noise is best for masking during pure tone air and bone conduction testing?**
   a. white noise
   b. speech noise
   c. narrow band noise
   d. broad band noise

4. **Effective masking may be described as:**
   a. an increased masking noise that does not shift the threshold tone
   b. a formula method to determine how much masking noise is appropriate
   c. a psychoacoustic method like the one proposed by Hood
   d. all of the above

5. **Masking is performed during air conduction testing when:**
   a. a 40 dB or more difference occurs between the air conduction threshold of the better ear and the poorer ear
   b. a 40 dB or more difference occurs between the air conduction threshold of the poorer ear and the bone conduction threshold of the better ear
   c. a 15 dB or more difference occurs between the air conduction threshold of the poorer ear and the bone conduction threshold of the better ear
   d. a and b

6. **Masking is performed during bone conduction testing whenever:**
   a. a 15 dB or more difference occurs between the obtained bone conduction threshold of the better ear and the obtained air conduction threshold of the poorer ear
   b. a 0 dB or more difference occurs between the obtained bone conduction threshold of the better ear and the obtained air conduction threshold of the poorer ear
   c. a 40 dB or more difference occurs between the obtained bone conduction threshold of the better ear and the obtained air conduction threshold of the poorer ear
   d. a and c

7. **The occlusion effect occurs during:**
   a. bone conduction testing causing thresholds to shift due to headphones being placed over the ear
   b. air conduction testing causing thresholds to shift due to headphones being placed over the ear
   c. impedance audiometry
   d. bone conduction testing causing threshold to shift due to the oscillator being placed on the skull

8. **A masking dilemma occurs when:**
   a. it is impossible to mask
   b. the patient displays a bilateral conductive loss
   c. masking can not be completed due to overmasking
   d. all of the above

9. **Undermasking is defined as:**
   a. occurring more often during air conduction testing
   b. occurring more often during bone conduction testing
   c. an excess of noise creating a false threshold
   d. masking noise being at least 40 dB above the true threshold

10. **Central masking can effect a threshold by:**
    a. 5 dB
    b. 20 dB
    c. 40 dB
    d. none of the above

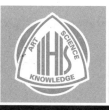
TEST INSTRUCTIONS

After you have finished reading this lesson, carefully study the selections from the **Required Reading.**

Then, look over the lesson once more to impress the important points on your memory.

When you are sure you know the lesson thoroughly, use the answer sheet in the back of the manual that corresponds to this lesson.

IMPORTANT: Place your student number on the answer sheets. Your student number appears on the inside front cover of the manual. **It must appear on your answer sheets in order for you to get credit for completion of the lesson.**

Once the answer sheet is completed, tear it out and mail to: International Institute for Hearing Instruments Studies
16880 Middlebelt Road, Suite 4, Livonia, MI 48154-3367

REQUIRED READING FOR THIS LESSON

Pages 60-65, 131-153, 168-175
Hearing Instrument Science and Fitting Practices (Second Edition)

TEST QUESTIONS

1. **In a sensorineural hearing loss, air conduction thresholds are:**
   a. better than bone conduction thresholds
   b. worse than bone conduction thresholds
   c. the same as bone conduction thresholds
   d. in normal range

2. **An air-bone gap means the:**
   a. air conduction thresholds are worse than bone conduction thresholds
   b. air conduction thresholds are better that bone conduction thresholds
   c. loss is purely conductive
   d. loss is purely mixed

3. **A sensorineural component is the difference between:**
   a. AC thresholds and the range of normal hearing
   b. BC thresholds and the range of normal hearing
   c. AC thresholds and BC thresholds
   d. BC thresholds and 0 dB HL

4. **A pure conductive loss shows:**
   a. all bone conduction thresholds within normal limits
   b. all air conduction thresholds out of normal range
   c. some bone conduction thresholds within normal limits
   d. a and b above

5. **In a purely conductive loss:**
   a. the inner ear nerve cells are impaired
   b. the outer or middle ear functions normally
   c. sound is reduced before its arrival at the inner ear
   d. nerve cells in the inner ear cannot respond readily to vibrations through the bones of the skull

6. **A mixed loss exhibits:**
   a. a sensorineural component
   b. a conductive component
   c. normal hearing by bone conduction
   d. a and b above

7. **An audiogram with less loss at the high and low frequencies than the middle frequency region is classified as a:**
   a. flat curve
   b. rising curve
   c. reverse slope
   d. trough-shaped curve

8. **Pure Tone Average estimates:**
   a. SRT
   b. the degree of difficulty in hearing
   c. the average of 250, 500 and 1000 Hz ÷ 3
   d. bone conduction thresholds

9. **To calculate PTA in a hearing loss when thresholds drop 15-20 dB or more at any or all frequencies:**
   a. add the 3 frequency thresholds and ÷ 3
   b. add the 2 frequencies with the most loss and ÷ 2
   c. add the 2 frequencies with the least loss and ÷ 2
   d. use 500 and 1000 Hz only and ÷ 2

10. **PTA describes the following audiogram classification fairly accurately:**
   a. flat loss
   b. fragmentary audiogram
   c. sudden drop
   d. a and b above

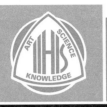
TEST INSTRUCTIONS

After you have finished reading this lesson, carefully study the selections from the **Required Reading.**

Then, look over the lesson once more to impress the important points on your memory.

When you are sure you know the lesson thoroughly, use the answer sheet in the back of the manual that corresponds to this lesson.

IMPORTANT: Place your student number on the answer sheets. Your student number appears on the inside front cover of the manual. **It must appear on your answer sheets in order for you to get credit for completion of the lesson.**

Once the answer sheet is completed, tear it out and mail to: International Institute for Hearing Instruments Studies
16880 Middlebelt Road, Suite 4, Livonia, MI 48154-3367

REQUIRED READING FOR THIS LESSON

Pages 93-102, 109-112
Hearing Instrument Science and Fitting Practices (Second Edition)

TEST QUESTIONS

1. **Although pure tones sound artificial to us, they have the advantage of:**
   a. being subjective
   b. measuring a specific frequency without involvement of other frequencies
   c. depending entirely of the patient's response and motivation
   d. using formulas as a substitute for speech tests

2. **Speech Reception Threshold:**
   a. like an audiogram, differs at each frequency
   b. is a level above SDT by about 8-10 dB
   c. proves useful when testing someone who does not speak English
   d. is always 20 dB for normal ears

3. **Dynamic Range is the usable range of hearing between:**
   a. SAT and MCL
   b. SRT and MCL
   c. SRT and UCL
   d. MCL and UCL

4. **The Most Comfortable Level is:**
   a. about 65 dB SPL for normal ears
   b. about 45 dB HL for normal ears
   c. the range of comfortable loudness
   d. a and b above

5. **The range between threshold and MCL:**
   a. forms a flat line across the audiogram
   b. is the same at each frequency
   c. differs at each frequency
   d. is a point on the HL dial, not frequency related

6. **A patient with a conductive loss has:**
   a. a wider dynamic range than normal ears
   b. the same dynamic range as normal ears
   c. a narrower dynamic range than normal ears
   d. a dynamic range that reduces by the amount of the conductive component

7. **When patients have a sensorineural loss, MCL:**
   a. retains a relationship with the lower boundary
   b. extends downward, affecting the lower boundary
   c. extends upward, increasing the dynamic range
   d. pushes UCL upward, raising the dynamic range

8. **Recruitment is:**
   a. common in patients with cochlear losses
   b. a result of a large conductive component making sound louder
   c. an abnormal increase in UCL
   d. an advantage when fitting high frequency losses

9. **When a patient has normal pure tone thresholds of 0 dB HL across frequencies, it is difficult to accurately measure:**
   a. SAT
   b. SRT
   c. MCL
   d. UCL

10. **When a patient has a large conductive component, it is difficult to accurately measure:**
    a. SAT
    b. SRT
    c. MCL
    d. UCL

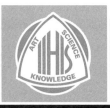
TEST INSTRUCTIONS

After you have finished reading this lesson, carefully study the selections from the **Required Reading.**

Then, look over the lesson once more to impress the important points on your memory.

When you are sure you know the lesson thoroughly, use the answer sheet in the back of the manual that corresponds to this lesson.

IMPORTANT: Place your student number on the answer sheets. Your student number appears on the inside front cover of the manual. **It must appear on your answer sheets in order for you to get credit for completion of the lesson.**

Once the answer sheet is completed, tear it out and mail to: International Institute for Hearing Instruments Studies
16880 Middlebelt Road, Suite 4, Livonia, MI 48154-3367

REQUIRED READING FOR THIS LESSON

Pages 112-114, 435-437, 798-836
Hearing Instrument Science and Fitting Practices (Second Edition)

TEST QUESTIONS

1. **Speech discrimination tests:**
    a. are easily understood at any level above SRT
    b. use spondiac words from single syllable word lists
    c. approximate a sample of speech sounds in an ordinary conversation
    d. contain redundancy unless they are too loud

2. **The patient has pure tone air conduction thresholds of 40 dB HL at each frequency.**
    If the patient has a conductive hearing loss, his MCL would be approximately:
    a. 60 dB HL or less
    b. 60-69 dB HL
    c. 70-79 dB HL
    d. 80 dB HL or above

3. **Discriminating complex sounds depend on:**
    a. redundancy
    b. timbre
    c. resonance
    d. frequency

4. **In a complex sound, the fundamental frequency is the:**
   a. harmonic
   b. loudest frequency
   c. overtone
   d. phoneme

5. **We recognize the different vowel sounds because of variations in:**
   a. the fundamental frequency
   b. overtones
   c. harmonics
   d. timbre

6. **A formant is:**
   a. a concentration of energy around certain frequencies
   b. the lowest frequency in a complex tone
   c. a weak, high frequency component or overtone
   d. a phoneme composed of several frequencies

7. **The most important energy for recognizing speech sounds are:**
   a. harmonics and overtones
   b. second and third formants
   c. the fundamental frequencies
   d. low frequency phonemes

8. **The upward spread of masking occurs when:**
   a. a low frequency sound masks out a high frequency sound
   b. a louder sound occurs immediately after a softer sound
   c. one sound follows another closely in time
   d. a high frequency sound is louder than a low frequency sound

9. **Masking is required for discrimination tests when:**
   a. masking was used for bone conduction tests
   b. masking was used for air conduction tests
   c. MCL's differ by 40 dB or more
   d. the discrimination test is conducted 40 dB above SRT

10. **Binaural testing:**
    a. helps decide which ear to fit
    b. is not important with similar audiograms
    c. is unnecessary when SRT, MCL and UCL are the same for both ears
    d. all of the above

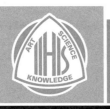
TEST INSTRUCTIONS

After you have finished reading this lesson, carefully study the selections from the **Required Reading.**

Then, look over the lesson once more to impress the important points on your memory.

When you are sure you know the lesson thoroughly, use the answer sheet in the back of the manual that corresponds to this lesson.

IMPORTANT: Place your student number on the answer sheets. Your student number appears on the inside front cover of the manual. **It must appear on your answer sheets in order for you to get credit for completion of the lesson.**

Once the answer sheet is completed, tear it out and mail to: International Institute for Hearing Instruments Studies
16880 Middlebelt Road, Suite 4, Livonia, MI 48154-3367

REQUIRED READING FOR THIS LESSON
Pages 122-124
Hearing Instrument Science and Fitting Practices (Second Edition)
Pages 68-73
Introduction to the Auditory System

TEST QUESTIONS

1. **Tympanometry identifies:**
    a. the hearing acuity of the patient
    b. a measure of the static compliance of the eustachean tube
    c. a measure of the dynamic compliance of the TM
    d. a measure of the central processing of the ear

2. **By convention, the range of pressures exerted in tympanometry range from:**
    a. +200mm (H20) to –200mm (H20)
    b. +400mm (H20) to –400mm (H20)
    c. +300mm (H20) to –300mm (H20)
    d. +100mm (H20) to –100mm (H20)

3. **The tympanogram measures:**
    a. the loudness of the sound
    b. the intensity of the sound in the cavity between the probe tip and the first bend of the canal
    c. the intensity of the sound in the cavity between the probe tip and the TM
    d. the spectrum of the sound in the cavity

4. **The point of maximum compliance in a tympanogram represents:**
   a. the absence of air pressure in the ear
   b. the point at which the pressure exerted through the probe tip exactly matches the pressure within the middle ear
   c. the point of best hearing thresholds
   d. the point of worst hearing thresholds

5. **A "0"mm (H20) pressure reading means:**
   a. that there is a vacuum in the cavity
   b. that the hearing acuity is within the range of normal limits
   c. that no pressure is being exerted on the TM
   d. that the pressure exerted matches the hearing loss

6. **Figure 14-3 represents what "Type" of tympanogram?**
   a. Type A
   b. Type As
   c. Type Ad
   d. Type B

7. **Figure 14-6 represents what "Type" of tympanogram?**
   a. Type A
   b. Type As
   c. Type Ad
   d. Type B

8. **Figure 14-7 represents what "Type" of tympanogram?**
   a. Type A
   b. Type As
   c. Type Ad
   d. Type C

9. **The configuration and height of the tympanogram can be a factor in deciding the proper matrix for the fitting of a hearing aid:**
   a. A Type B tells us to decrease the output by 5 dB
   b. A Type C tells us to increase the output by 20 dB
   c. A Type C tells us to decrease the output by 15 dB
   d. A high Type A tells us to decrease the output by 2–3 dB

10. **Tympanometry is effective in identifying:**
    a. middle ear pathologies
    b. cochlear pathologies
    c. VIIIth Cranial nerve pathologies
    d. all of the above

INTERNATIONAL INSTITUTE FOR HEARING INSTRUMENTS STUDIES

DISTANCE LEARNING for Professionals in HEARING HEALTH SCIENCES

IIHIS

Unit III - Hearing Instruments

CONTENTS

The lessons in this unit explain Sound Pressure Level (SPL) measurements for hearing instruments, hearing instrument selection, electronics and history, rationale for fitting (CIC) hearing aids and digital technology.

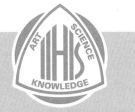

Published by
International Institute for Hearing Instruments Studies
Educational Division of International Hearing Society

ACOUSTICS

It is relatively easy to measure where a patient starts to hear, what is comfortable, and when sound becomes too loud. Fitting a hearing aid requires us to alter or change the sound in some way, boosting one frequency or eliminating another. To do this efficiently, we require more information on the properties of sound, how to measure it, and how the patient perceives it.

Sound is a form of energy. Sound originates only when another form of energy creates a vibration in the molecules of a solid, liquid or gas. When anything vibrates, it has organized back and forth movement. Movement involves speed, distance and time. These are some of the physical attributes of sound.

The human ear, however, perceives sound as something quite different. Our sensory input judges sound by its loudness, pitch and timbre or tonal quality, all psychological attributes, differing from one person to another.

Acoustics, the branch of physics specializing in sound, has two sub-fields relating to human hearing - Physiological Acoustics and Psychological Acoustics.

PHYSIOLOGICAL ACOUSTICS

This field covers any physical aspect of sound precisely measured with instruments. Consider these 'the laws,' if you will.

Physical Definition of Sound. Sound is a propagated change or disturbance in the density, and therefore in the pressure, of an elastic medium.

A propagated change or disturbance involves a vibrating body, and for our purposes, the elastic medium is almost always air. The medium can be a gas, a solid, or a liquid. Sound cannot travel through a vacuum.

Any medium consists of molecules in a position of rest. A vibrating body causes these molecules to vibrate back and forth at the same rate as the vibrating body.

As molecules in air remain unseen, let's use a different example. Line up ten people (molecules), shoulder to shoulder, with 1" separating each of them (in a position of rest). You, the vibrating body, push the shoulder of the first person (molecule) toward the others. A chain reaction occurs. Each person hits the next person, then bounces back. Some people are pushed together while others are inches apart until they return to their normal position of

rest. You have created a wave of vibrating motion. The wave travelled. The people did not. They returned to their position of rest.

Sound travels in waves. Only the waves travel, the air does not. Sound waves travel in expanding spheres or 'shells' in all directions. These spheres are **longitudinal waves,** travelling in the same direction as the vibrating body.

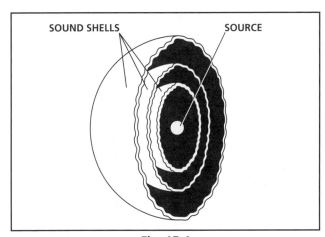

Fig. 15-1
Sound Waves

The chief sources of sound waves are:

1. a vibrating body, such as a tuning fork, loudspeaker diaphragm, or violin string, and

2. a throttled or modified airstream, like a siren, a clarinet or the human voice.

When the wave travels, some of the air molecules are pushed together - compression, others are farther apart than normal - rarefaction. A complete sound wave has an area of compression and of rarefaction.

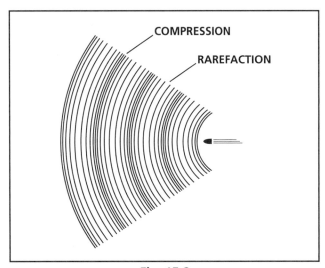

Fig. 15-2
Compression & Rarefaction in Four Complete Sound Waves

If we strike a tuning fork, the prongs of the fork vibrate back and forth, producing sound waves of compression and rarefaction. We cannot see sound waves, although we know the tuning fork vibrates. If we attach a pen to one prong of the tuning fork, and move a sheet of paper beneath the pen, we produce a series of wavy lines on the paper, corresponding to the vibrations of compression and rarefaction.

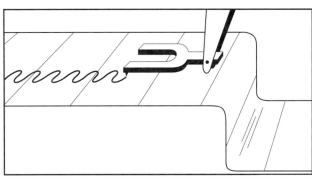

Fig. 15-3
Tuning Fork Producing a Sine Wave

Sine Waves: A **tone** is a sound sensation with a stable or fairly stable pitch. A tuning fork produces **pure tones,** with simple, uncomplicated alternations of compression and rarefaction, **sine waves.** The vertical axis of the wavy line shows the **amplitude or loudness of the wave.** The

horizontal axis records the **time** elapsed. The amplitude varies with the force applied to make the tuning fork vibrate. More force increases the amplitude, and therefore the time required to cease vibration.

Frequency: The number of times a vibrating body completes a pattern of complete cycles of compression and rarefaction per second is the frequency of that sound wave.

Frequency is measured in cycles per second, or Hertz. These terms are often shortened to kilohertz, especially in the higher frequencies. All of the following equal 2000 Hz.

| 2000 Hz | 2000 cps | 2 kcs | 2 kHz |

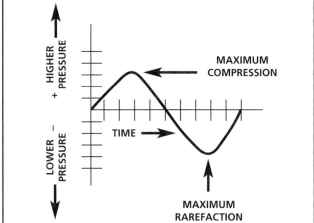

Fig. 15-4
One Cycle

The graph above represents one cycle, a complete alternation from normal pressure at zero, to maximum compression, back through zero, to maximum rarefaction, and back again to zero. One cycle completes one compression and one rarefaction. One complete cycle is 360°, like a circle.

From zero to maximum

amplitude in compression is	90°
Back to zero	90°
To maximum rarefaction	90°
To zero again	90°
Total	360°

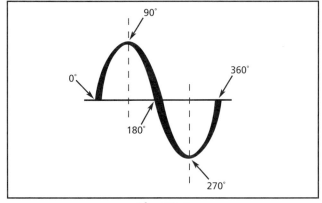

Fig. 15-5
One Cycle in Degrees

Period: A period is the time required for one complete cycle of compression and rarefaction, represented on the horizontal axis.

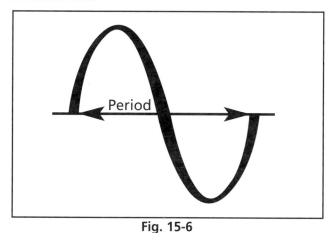

Fig. 15-6
One Period

For example, a 250 Hz tone vibrates 250 cycles in one second. The period of time taken for one complete cycle is

Period = $\dfrac{1}{\text{Frequency}}$

Period = $\dfrac{1}{250}$ or 1.000 divided by 250

Period = .004 seconds or 4 milliseconds

An 8000 Hz tone, vibrating 8000 times per second, has a much shorter period.

Period = $\dfrac{1}{8000}$ or 1.000 divided by 8000

Period = .000125 seconds or 125 microseconds.

Frequency and Amplitude. Amplitude graphically describes the **Intensity** of the energy a vibrating body delivers. Intensity is usually expressed in dB.

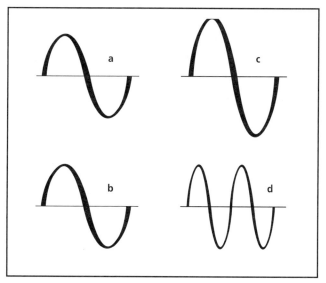

Fig. 15-7
Frequency and Amplitude

Compare the 1 Hz sine waves, 'a' and 'c', in Fig. 15-7. Both have the same period, but 'c' has greater amplitude or intensity.

Sine waves 'b' and 'd' have the same amplitude, but 'd' has two areas of compression and rarefaction in the same period of time, **double the frequency.**

If sine wave 'b' is 1 Hz, then 'd' is 2 Hz.

Speed of Sound, Velocity: Sound waves travel in air at about **1,100 feet per second,** or 340 meters per second, or more than 760 miles per hour. A supersonic airplane 'breaking the sound barrier' exceeds this speed.

Sound travels about four times faster through water, and fourteen times faster through steel, than air. Have you ever listened for a train with your ear to the rail? You hear the train coming through the steel rail before you hear it through the air.

All sounds, regardless of frequency, travel at the same speed, or velocity, which, for our purposes is 1,100'/second in air. The distance a high-frequency sound covers in one second is the same as the distance covered by a low-frequency sound. The distance **per cycle, or wavelength** of a high frequency sound is shorter, but the shorter wavelength has more cycles in the same period of time.

Wavelength: Wavelength is the distance covered by one complete cycle of a wave. You can start from zero or any other degree along the wave, as long as you measure to the same degree on the next wave.

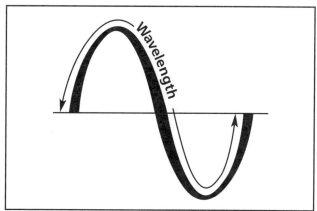

Fig. 15-8
Wavelength

In 'b' of Fig. 15-7, one wavelength is the distance from the beginning of the sine wave to the end, from zero, including both compression and rarefaction, to zero again. In 'd', one wavelength is from the beginning of the sine wave, through one compression and rarefaction, to zero. The wavelength of 'd' is **half as long** as 'b'.

In other words, 'd' is double the frequency and half the wavelength of 'b'.

Wavelength, Frequency and Velocity: The wavelength, frequency and velocity of sound are inter-related. Again, let's use 250 Hz and 8000 Hz as examples for comparison.

$$\text{FREQUENCY} = \frac{\text{VELOCITY}}{\text{WAVELENGTH}}$$

250 Hz $250 = \dfrac{1100'/\text{sec}}{\text{Wavelength}}$

or 250 wavelengths =   1100'
    1 wavelength =   4.4' (1100 divided by 250)

8000 Hz $8000 = \dfrac{1100'/\text{sec}}{\text{Wavelength}}$

or 8000 wavelengths =   1100' (1100 divided by 8000)
      1 wavelength =   .1375' or (times 12) 1.65 inches.

If you double the frequency, you half the distance of the wavelength. Let's see if this works.

250 Hz	=	4.4'
500 Hz	=	2.2'
1000 Hz	=	1.1'
2000 Hz	=	0.55' or 6.6 inches
4000 Hz	=	0.275' or 3.3 inches
8000 Hz	=	0.1375' or 1.65 inches

How long would a wavelength of 125 Hz be?

$4.4 \times 2 = 8.8'$

Temperature: Sound travels faster through a medium with a higher temperature. For example, sound travels in air at 340 meters per second when the temperature is 20° C, 72° F. At a lower temperature, 0° C, 32° F (freezing point), sound travels at about 330 meters per second.

Reflection: Reflection is a characteristic of sound and light. Sound reflects more from a flat, hard surface than from an uneven or porous surface. Sounds reflecting from the walls, floor, or ceiling of a room are **reverberations,** leaving a persistence of sound after the sound ceases. An **echo** is a sound reflection, heard separately from the original sound.

Absorption: The opposite of reflection is absorption. Draperies, carpets, or upholstered furniture absorb sound waves and reduce reflections and echoes. Even air, itself, absorbs (attenuates) sound. The amount of absorption depends on moisture content and temperature.

SOUND PRESSURE

When sound waves travel, the **air pressure** in the compression part of the wave is slightly higher than normal, and slightly below normal when the molecules are more separated during rarefaction.

Sound pressure is the difference between the actual pressure at any point in a sound wave at any instant, and the average pressure at that point.

A sine wave is a wave of only one frequency. If another tone of the same frequency is added to our sine wave, then the pressure changes to accommodate the added wave. How these tones combine depends on phase.

Phase: When a sound wave begins at 0° or ends at 360°, it is **in phase.** Two tones of the **same frequency,** presented simultaneously - in phase - combine the pressures, causing higher compression and lower rarefaction. This combination gives the wave greater amplitude or volume. **You hear one louder tone.**

Phase can also mean the direction or location of the sound source as compared to the position of the listener, using 360° around the listener, with 0° or 360° being dead center. This is the concept for binaural hearing. Each ear hears the same input simultaneously. They fuse together, making the combined input appear louder.

When the sound reaches one ear before the other, **slightly out of phase, we determine direction,** and can locate the source of the sound. Our sense of direction, then, is because two identical sounds reach each ear slightly out of phase.

When two tones of **almost identical frequency,** i.e. 1000 Hz and 1003 Hz combine, you hear a noticeable increase and decrease, **a beat,** in the tone three times a second. This beat is **the difference in frequency. You hear a 1000 Hz tone and the beats.**

As the difference in frequency increases, i.e., 1005 Hz, 1009 Hz, the beats per second increase, changing to a pulse, then a roughness. When the difference between the two frequencies becomes large enough, you hear a third tone, the **difference tone,** as well as the higher and lower tone. The difference tone, measured in Hz, is the difference between the two frequencies, i.e., 1000 Hz, 1050 Hz, and 50 Hz.

Two tones of the **same frequency and intensity,** presented **180° out of phase cancel each other** out. The higher compression pressure of the first wave is reduced by the lower rarefaction pressure on the second wave. This occurs on each half of the wave. **You hear nothing.**

Complex Wave: A complex wave is made up of several different combined pure tones. Whenever you introduce more than one tone, the pressure interaction depends on the frequency, intensity and phase of each wave. Each instantaneous amplitude of the combined waves add together or fully or partially cancel each other out.

Periodic Waves: Some complex sounds, like music, or many sounds of speech, repeat themselves smoothly over time. These sounds are **periodic.**

Aperiodic Waves: Other sounds contain random complex tones without a period or pattern. These **aperiodic** sounds are usually perceived as noise.

Sound Power: Power is a characteristic of sound. A vibrating body, like a tuning fork, **forces** the air molecules to move back and forth. When these air pressure changes are measured in watts/cm^2, the force or power is **Intensity Level (IL).**

Pressure is generated whenever a force is applied to a surface area. Sound power transforms (transduces) into sound pressure when it touches a receiver, like the tympanic membrane or a microphone.

Sound pressure changes in sound waves are extremely small, - too small, for instance, to be measured in pounds per square inch, like atmospheric pressure at 14.7 lbs. per square inch.

Effective Sound Pressure: Microbar or one dyne per square centimeter is the basic unit for measuring sound pressure. It represents the amount of **energy** required to move a mass of one gram a distance of one centimeter in one second. In pressure, it equals one millionth of normal atmospheric pressure at sea level. One square centimeter covers an area of 0.0001 meters.

Weakest Sound: The weakest sound that **average, normal young ears** can hear, in the **best listening conditions,** in the most sensitive frequency range of the ear, is an **effective sound pressure of about two ten-thousandths dyne per square centimeter (0.0002 dyne/cm^2),** spoken as 'point triple-oh two dyne per square centimeter'.

The smallest audible power to create this pressure is 0.0000000000000001 watts. (10^{-16} watts/cm^2).

Strongest Sound: The strongest sound **normal** human ears can tolerate is at an **effective sound pressure of about 1,000 dynes/cm^2,** just below the threshold of pain. Sound pressure at 2000 dyne/cm^2, equal to a power of .01 watts/cm^2, (10^{-2} watts/cm^2), may damage the ear.

An enormous range of values exist between the weakest and strongest sound pressures. In fact, if the lower limit (0.0002) equals one, the upper limit of this range would equal 5,000,000. The loudest sound we can tolerate does not sound five million times as loud as the weakest sound we can hear.

Reference Levels: The effective sound pressure standard reference level of 0.0002 dynes/cm^2 approximates the point between silence and hearing for **normal human ears** in the middle range of audible frequencies.

This reference level is equal to 10^{-16} watts/cm^2, the IL reference level.

Effective sound pressure is measured in dynes per square centimeter (**0.0002 dynes/cm^2**), or **0.0002 microbar** in the centimeter-kilogram-second system. The meter-kilogram-second system uses **20 micro Newtons per square meter** or **20 micro Pascals. All four measurements are identical.** As most of the required reading uses 0.0002 dynes/cm^2, we will use this term throughout the lessons.

Decibel: Because of the problems of working with such a vast range of values in effective sound pressure, Alexander Graham Bell developed the **decibel, a tenth of a Bel.** This logarithmic scale translates the range of 0.0002 to 2,000 into a range of 0 to 140 dB.

The **logarithmic scale** reduces large numbers to the **base of ten, giving them the number 10 and an exponent.**

For example, $100 = 10 \times 10$ or 10^2
$1,000 = 10 \times 10 \times 10$ or 10^3
$100,000 = 10 \times 10 \times 10 \times 10 \times 10$ or 10^5

Counting the zeros is the easiest way to find the exponent.

When a number has a **minus exponent,** there is a **decimal point, followed by zeros, then 1.** For example, the smallest audible power is 0.000000000000001 watts/cm^2, 15 zeros after the decimal point, then 1, a total of 16 places after the decimal. The logarithmic method is 10^{-16} watts/cm^2.

You can see why an exponent is easier to handle.

A **Bel** is a ratio of two intensities, expressed 10:1.

1 Bel	=	10: 1
2 Bels	=	100: 1
3 Bels	=	1000: 1

A **decibel** is one-tenth of a bel. The decibel is a **ratio** between **two pressures (SPL)** or **two powers (IL).** It has **no fixed absolute value.**

For instance, increasing **one decibel** from 140 to 141 dB SPL increases the absolute pressure **10 million times more** than increasing from 0 dB SPL to 1 dB SPL. Normal ears can **just notice a difference (jnd)** in 3-4 dB SPL at very faint levels, but the jnd for very intense sound is 0.3 dB SPL.

Decibels measure **Power, in Intensity Level (IL),** expressed in watts, and **Pressure, in Sound Pressure Level (SPL),** expressed in dynes. The **power standard reference level of 10^{-16} Watts/cm^2 equals 0.0002 dynes/cm^2.** Intensity Level (IL) means we compare a power output in watts/cm^2

to the power reference level of 10^{-16} watts/cm^2, and express our answer in dB IL.

Sound Pressure Level (SPL) compares the effective sound pressure you are using in dynes/cm^2 to the reference level of 0.0002 dynes/cm^2, and expresses the answer in dB SPL.

Intensity and pressure are two different ways of looking at the same sound wave. They are directly related. The formula is

$\quad$ I = P^2 $\qquad$ Intensity equals Pressure squared.

To square a number, multiply the number by itself, i.e., 100 x 100 = 10,000 or 10^4, or multiply its log by 2. $(10^2)^2 = 10^4$.

The formula for calculating decibels in Intensity Level (IL) is:

dB IL = 10 log 10 $\underline{\text{Power A}}$
$\qquad\qquad\qquad$ Power B (reference level of 10^{-16} watts/cm^2)

If I = P^2, then we must multiply the log by 2 to have a pressure formula.

dB SPL = 10 x 2 x log 10 $\underline{\text{Pressure A}}$
$\qquad\qquad\qquad$ Pressure B
$\qquad\qquad$ (reference level of 0.0002 dynes/cm^2)

Since 10 x 2 = 20, our formula now becomes

dB SPL = 20 log 10 $\underline{\text{Pressure A}}$
$\qquad\qquad\qquad$ Pressure B (ref. level of 0.0002 dynes/cm^2)

Let's use an example for this procedure. We measure a sound, and find a pressure of 0.02 dyne/cm^2. This measured sound becomes Pressure A, the numerator in our formula; and the standard reference level is Pressure B, the denominator. Our equation now looks like this:

$\qquad$ dB = 20 log 10 $\qquad\qquad$ .02
$\qquad\qquad\qquad\qquad\qquad\qquad$ .0002

In simple English, this formula says 'divide .0002 into .02, and express this answer in a base 10 log with an exponent. Multiply the exponent by 20.

Dividing .0002 into .02 gives us 100.

dB = 20 log 10 100 (100 is 10^2 - Use exponent only)

dB = 20 x 2

dB = 40

This is a simple example. When the measured sound is not an exact multiple of the reference level, you must work the logarithm out in detail, or refer to a table of logarithms.

Fortunately, we do not complete this mathematical calculation. Audiometers and hearing instrument specifications do the job for us.

If I = P^2 and we know the pressure in dB SPL, then we can calculate dB IL by dividing by 2. To convert dB IL to SPL, multiply by 2.

dB IL	dB SPL
3	6
10	20
20	40
30	60
50	100

COMBINING SOUND from DIFFERENT SOURCES

The decibel is a calculated ratio. Decibels cannot be added together or subtracted, except exponentially.

When the sound pressure is doubled, the dB value is not. You must convert to dyne/cm^2, then **add** the pressures.

When we test the patient in competing noise, we measure each sound source separately, not the combination of the two sounds together. For example, if discrimination words are 60 dBA and noise is 60 dBA, then the signal to noise ratio (S/N) is 1:1, and the combined output is 66 dB.

When SPL values are doubled, the number of decibels increases by 6 dB.

When a power value (IL) is doubled, the number of decibels increases by 3 dB.

Because dB is a ratio that does not have an absolute or fixed value, it always has a reference level. Reference levels are as follows:

dB IL	10^{-16} watt/cm^2
dB SPL	0.0002 dyne/cm^2
dB HL	Audiometric Zero - ANSI Standards
dB SL	The Patient's threshold

COMPARISON of ANSI, ISO and ASA STANDARDS

Audiometer Frequency in Hz	dB of Pressure Above 20 Micro Newtons/Meter^2		
	ANSI (1969)	ISO (1964)	ASA (1951)
250	25.5	24.5	39.5
500	11.5	11.0	25.0
1000	7.0	6.5	16.5
2000	9.0	8.5	17.0
4000	9.5	9.0	15.0
8000	13.0	9.5	21.0

Fig. 15-9 Comparison of ANSI, ISO and ASA Standards

Each of the numbers in Fig. 15-9 represented **0 dB HL** on the audiogram. Use of older audiograms requires that you also know the standard the audiometer was calibrated to meet. This information usually appears on the audiogram.

Again, it is extremely important to use the letters SPL, IL, HL or SL to identify what kind of dB you are using.

COMPARISON of IL and SPL

	IL				SPL	
	Power				Pressure	
Watt/cm^2	Power Ratio	dB IL	dB SPL		Pressure Ratio	Dyne/cm^2
10^{-2}	100,000,000,000,000:1	70	140		10,000,000:1	2000.
10^{-3}	10,000,000,000,000:1	65	130		3,160,000:1	632.
10^{-4}	1,000,000,000,000:1	60	120		1,000,000:1	200.
10^{-5}	100,000,000,000:1	55	110		316,000:1	63.2
10^{-6}	10,000,000,000:1	50	100		100,000:1	20.
10^{-7}	1,000,000,000:1	45	90		31,600:1	6.32
10^{-8}	100,000,000:1	40	80		10,000:1	2.0
10^{-9}	10,000,000:1	35	70		3,160:1	0.632
10^{-10}	1,000,000:1	30	60		1,000:1	0.2
10^{-11}	1000,000:1	25	50		316:1	0.0632
10^{-12}	10,000:1	20	40		100:1	0.02
10^{-13}	1,000:1	15	30		31.6:1	0.00632
10^{-14}	100:1	10	20		10:1	0.002
10^{-15}	10:1	5	10		3.16:1	0.000632
10^{-16}	Reference Level 1:1	0	0	Reference Level 1:1		0.0002

For example in the highlighted box above:

$$\frac{I = P^2}{I = P}$$
$$\frac{I = 3.16 \times 3.16 = 10:1}{10 = 3.16:1}$$

dB IL x 2 = dB SPL   5 x 2 = 10 dB SPL

dB SPL ÷ 2 = dB IL   10 ÷ 2 = 5 dB IL

Zero dB does not mean the absence of sound. It means the amount of sound pressure you are comparing is equal to the reference level – and no pressure increase occurs.

Psychological acoustics includes everything that can be perceived by the human ear from a sensory standpoint - how sound 'feels' to us. Psychological acoustics requires a human ear.

What we measure as frequency, the ear perceives as pitch. Intensity measurements we interpret as loudness, timbre as tonal quality.

Intensity and Loudness: Intensity, measured in dB IL, SPL or HL is a physical measurement. Other words that describe intensity are amplitude and Maximum Sound Pressure. Loudness is psychological. We perceive a small increase in the intensity of a soft sound as a significant increase in loudness. We require a greater change in intensity to make a loud sound louder than to make a soft sound louder.

If we make a sound twice as intense, we would expect it to be twice as loud. This is not the case. Most auditory systems follow a **power law,** sometimes considered a **logarithmic concept,** because a **10 dB increase doubles the loudness** over most of the range of intensities. We already know that when we double the sound pressure or intensity, a 6 dB increase occurs. A threefold increase in sound pressure, 10 dB, doubles the loudness. For example, a 1000 Hz pure tone at 80 dB SPL is twice as loud as 70 dB SPL, and half as loud as 90 dB SPL.

Loudness level across frequencies is measured in phons. Loudness, up frequency, uses sones for measurement.

Phons: **Phons compare the loudness level** of a sound at one frequency to the same loudness at another frequency. Although the loudness is the same, the intensity required varies at each frequency. **The loudness level reference point in phons is 40 dB SPL at 1000 Hz equals 40 phons.** The phon graph in Lesson 7 shows how normal ears perceive sound. The following graph typifies a sensorineural loss.

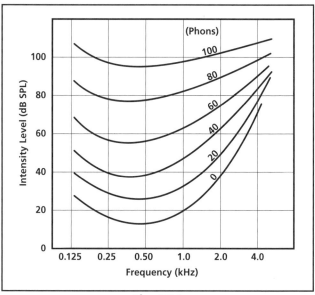

Fig. 16-1
Sensorineural Loss in Phons

Here, the lower frequencies grow faster than the mid frequencies, but higher frequencies notice a greater change in loudness when the increase is only a few dB.

Recruitment exemplifies both the physical and psychological meanings of intensity and loudness. A small increase in the physical measurement in dB appears to be a large increase in subjective loudness. Although the two meanings are related, the relationship changes from one person to another.

Sones: Another unit of subjective loudness, the **sone,** uses average normal judgements of **loudness going up frequency,** not across frequency. **One sone equals a 1000 Hz tone at 40 dB SPL,** which, for normal ears is also 40 phons. Above 40 phons, or 1 sone, a 10 phon increase in loudness doubles the loudness to two sones.

Sound grows quicker above a sensation level of 40 dB for a normal auditory system. An average sensation level to MCL in normal ears is 40 dB. If phon lines match sones for normal ears above MCL, then we should expect sensorineural losses to also have greater loudness growth above MCL. This is why the Forced Choice Method of finding MCL works so well.

Frequency and Pitch: **Frequency and Pitch** also share this kind of relationship. Frequency, the physical measurement in Hz, or cycles per second, relates to the listeners interpretation of pitch, the phychological measurement of whether a sound is low or high. Raising the frequency of a sound makes the pitch higher. Doubling the frequency raises the pitch one octave, but does not double the pitch.

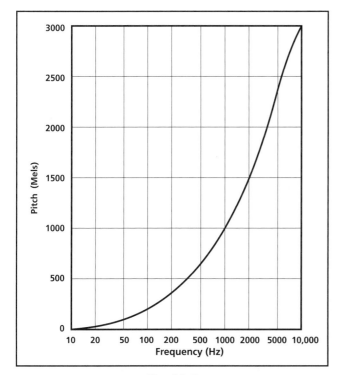

Fig. 16-2
Mel Scale

Mels measure pitch. 1000 Mels is the pitch of a 1000 Hz tone at a 40 dB sensation level, MCL for normal ears. A higher pitched sound will have more mels, a lower pitched sound, less.

For example, doubling the frequency (the definition of one octave) from 1000 Hz to 2000 Hz changes the pitch of a 40 dB SL tone from 1000 mels (the reference point for mels) to 1500 mels. If the pitch doubled too, 2000 Hz would be 2000 mels, but a pitch of 2000 mels is not reached until about 3000 Hz.

The subjective loudness of a sound relates to pitch, sensation level and the type of hearing loss. The duration of the sound also plays a part. For example, a person with auditory fatigue (tone decay) perceives the sound as getting quieter. As the sound gets quieter, the pitch changes too.

Critical Bands: Normal ears really don't detect a difference between 1 mel and 2 mels or 20 mels and 30 mels. Relatively narrow bands of nearly the same frequency become one pitch. In the mid frequencies, the narrow **critical bands** are about 100 mels or 1/3 octave wide at normal loudness levels. There are 22 critical bands between 20 Hz and 9300 Hz.

Some critical bands become abnormally widened in an impaired cochlea, giving the hearing impaired person **reduced frequency resolution.**

Critical bands are like frequency filters, or a 'Fourier Spectral Analysis of the cochlea'. For example, normal hearing easily discriminates a 1000 Hz tone from a 1030 Hz tone, a 3% change. But, a grossly distorted ear may find no difference between 1000 Hz and 1500 Hz.

A widened critical band reduces the patient's ability to detect some necessary frequency components in a complex sound, like music or speech. It may not be possible for the patient to hear the difference between certain letter combinations, like 'ith' and 'if'. Widened critical bands are one of the factors contributing to the reduced ability of cochlear losses to hear in background noise.

The physically measured loudness of a sound includes frequency, intensity, and duration. These measurements remain constant regardless of whether hearing is normal, conductive, mixed or sensorineural. Although the measurements remain fixed, they are perceived differently by each patient because of the type of individual hearing loss.

SPEECH

Our speech tests, so far, relate to listening to someone else talk. With normal hearing, we automatically monitor our own speech in several ways.

1. We hear our own voice, automatically correcting ourselves if we pronounce any letter or word incorrectly.

2. We raise our voice in the presence of background noise so that we can continue to monitor our voice.

3. We raise our voice when speaking to someone at a distance.

4. When conversing in a quiet room, we lower our voice automatically.

5. We hear our voice from both the inside, by bone conduction, and through our ears. For instance, a 'v' vibrates air on our bottom lip and front teeth. We feel it and hear it at the lip. An 'rrr' feels like it is formed at the throat and we hear it coming from the same spot.

6. When we get a bad cold, our voice is affected. We have trouble forming certain words, like 'plum jam'. We know our mouth moved properly, but our ears hear 'blub jab'.

Our voice feels like it's trapped inside our neck and chest. Yet, all we have is a temporary, mild, conductive loss.

We know that speech production changes in a number of ways when serious permanent hearing loss occurs.

A person with a sudden loss, like mumps or meningitis, maintains speech for a short time, then it deteriorates rapidly.

The speech of a patient with a gradual loss, like presbycusis or otosclerosis, deteriorates slowly as the hearing loss progresses. First, the quieter high frequency sounds like s, sh, ch, f, or th, become distorted or omitted. Consonants at the end of words slur. Voice quality changes, sounding more mechanical, and the patient is unable to control the volume of their voice in certain situations as the hearing deteriorates.

Most hearing loss is gradual. The way you hear yourself today does not sound any different from the way you heard yourself yesterday. You have no way to compare your voice to a year ago, or five years ago. The change is so subtle and gradual that **your perception of normal changes** to match what you hear, and there is no awareness of change.

If the letter 's' no longer whistles, it sounds more like a slur, then you pronounce it this way over time. You recognize when you have difficulty discriminating others, but **your voice always sounds normal to you.**

You will hear a patient describe their voice as 'gravelly, now that I'm getting older'. The patient judges the quality of their voice based on age, but does not associate it with hearing because it sounds the same today as it did yesterday, or last week.

A person with acquired unilateral loss remarks that they no longer have a sense of direction - and the volume of speech in others is quieter, or they cannot monitor the volume of their own voice as well. It is obvious, when masking the better ear for speech tests, that they have not lost all of their ability to monitor the volume of their own voice. As soon as you introduce the masking noise, the volume of their voice increases considerably - **the Lombard effect.** This effect does not happen with masking in the poorer ear.

Anyone faking (malingering) hearing loss will increase the volume of their own voice in the presence of masking, but genuine hearing loss continues to speak at the same level as before.

A person with normal hearing judges their speech by the way it sounds. A deaf child is taught how to make this judgement by the way it feels. Because normal hearing can hear the sounds, we really don't give much thought to the way it feels, except during short intervals like a bad cold, when the 'feeling' is disrupted.

Neither does a person with gradual hearing loss. But, one thing is certain. **If you change the way they hear, you are going to change the way they hear themselves.** A hearing instrument helps to raise many of the elements of their own speech, inaudible before amplification, to a usable level. Prepare the patient for this change.

SPEECH PRODUCTION

When we speak, the larynx pushes air from the lungs through open or closed vocal cords and creates the **fundamental frequency** in our voice. This fundamental frequency falls between 120 and 250 Hz in men, and 210 to 325 Hz in women.

The vocal folds set up secondary vibrations, **harmonics,** which reinforce some frequencies more than others. The reinforced frequencies are **formants.** We form the vowels and consonants with this air, using our mouth, lips, tongue, and teeth. This causes the formants to change, but they are independent of the fundamental frequency in our voice.

We use either **voicing** or **articulated sounds** to form each phoneme.

Voicing is the noise the air makes as it passes through the vocal cords, like 'oh' and 'aye', while articulated sounds control the air with the tongue, like 'k', teeth, like 's', or lips, like 'p'.

Vowels use more open vocal cord voicing, have more low frequency energy and volume, and tend to take longer over time than consonants. We feel more vibration or resonance with any voiced sound, regardless of whether the vocal cords are open or closed.

Resonant consonants include m, n, ing, w, y, l, and r.

Articulation sounds have higher frequency energy, and less volume and vibration because the air is controlled through the lips, tongue or teeth.

This process is natural, and hard to reverse. Try to say 'teach' with the 't' sound loudest and the 'e' sound quietest.

Just because a sound is louder does not mean that speech is more intelligible, or the loud sounds give a better basis for understanding. If that were the case, then we would be able to estimate a sentence with only vowel sounds.

_____e _oe _ou_ _i.

Consonants cannot give the total meaning either.

Th_ sh_ sh_ld f_t.

We need a balance between both the vowels and consonants for intelligibility. We also require **formant transitions,** where the vocal cords are beginning to form the next phoneme by moving energy peaks to other frequency regions within the vocal tract. If we use only the sound of the letters shown in the above sentences, our mouth is not in the right position to form the next letter. We require a formant transition to accomplish this task. With vowels, formant transitions and consonants present, the sentence is very easy to interpret or repeat.

The shoe should fit.

The average levels of speech, measured in front of the lips at a distance of one meter (3') are:

Average Male Speaker	65 dB SPL
Average Female Speaker	63 dB SPL
Talking as loud as possible	85 dB SPL
Talking as soft as possible	45 dB SPL
Range of whisper to shout	40 dB SPL

Although the average level is 65 dB SPL, the fluctuation to allow for the loudest and softest sounds in conversational speech is ± 12 dB, giving the loudest speech sounds an intensity of 65 + 12 = 77 dB.

One way of looking at the relationship between loudness and clarity is a comparison of power and intelligibility within each frequency range.

POWER and INTELLIGIBILITY

FREQUENCY RANGE (Hz)	PER CENT SPEECH POWER	PER CENT INTELLIGIBILITY
62 –125	5 ⎫	1 ⎫
125 – 250	13 ⎬ 60	1 ⎬ 5
250 – 500	42 ⎭ ⎫ 95	3 ⎭
500 – 1000	35 ⎭	35 ⎫
1000 – 2000	3 ⎫	35 ⎪
2000 – 4000	1 ⎬ 5	13 ⎬ 60 ⎫ 95
4000 – 8000	1 ⎭	12 ⎭

Fig. 16-3
Comparison Chart

We know that vowels are louder than consonants, and they contain more low frequencies than consonants. This excess of low frequency power is not advantageous in the understanding of speech.

If we eliminate all the power below 500 Hz, we lose only 5% of the intelligibility. If we eliminate all the power above 1000 Hz, we lose 5% of the power and 60% of the intelligibility. The area of 500 - 1000 Hz is pretty evenly balanced at 35% for both power and intelligibility.

Other research expresses this concept in a different way.

POWER and CLARITY

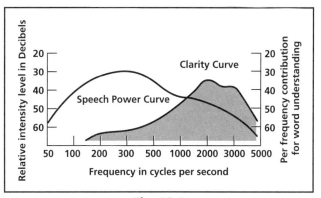

Fig. 16-4
The Speech Power Curve
and the Speech Clarity Curve

Power is referenced on the left in decibels; clarity is referenced on the right in perfrequency contribution for word understanding.

This graph shows a greater concentration of power in the lower frequency vowel area, with a tapering off through the higher frequency consonants.

We filter away frequencies until we have the best clarity for speech. We need the higher frequencies for clarity but have very little volume or power. Power in the lower frequency vowel area gives the voice timbre and tonal quality, as well as clarity in the higher frequencies.

The American National Standards Institute (ANSI) developed the **Articulation Index (AI),** expressing clarity in percent as follows:

250 Hz	8%
500 Hz	14%
1000 Hz	22%
2000 Hz	33%
4000 Hz	23%

SPEECH CIRCUIT of AUDIOMETER

When our patient chooses MCL on the audiometer, the choice is based on a 'flat' frequency response, with the judgement of loudness based on the volume in the 1000 Hz area.

Adjusting the volume in dB raises or lowers this flat response. No area is over or under emphasized. For example, our patient chooses MCL at 65 dB HL. To convert this speech level to SPL, using ANSI Standards, we add 20 dB. The MCL in SPL is 85 dB.

However, the patient hears this speech through earphones. As the ear canals are not plugged, ear canal resonance enhances this speech.

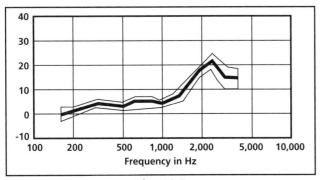

Fig. 16-5
Ear Canal Resonance Response

Let's assume that 0 on the left side of the graph is now 85. The ear canal resonance boosts the higher frequencies by as much as 25 dB around 2700 Hz!

When fitting a hearing instrument, either the instrument itself, or an earmold blocks off the ear canal. This loss of ear canal resonance is **insertion loss.** The patient also has the occlusion effect, where their own voice appears louder.

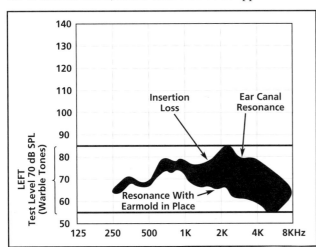

Fig. 16-6
Insertion Loss

We must compensate for insertion loss and reduce the occlusion effect.

EFFECTS of EARMOLDS on FREQUENCY RESPONSE

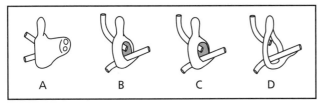

Fig. 16-7
Earmolds

Each of the above earmolds has tubing to input sound, like hooking up a 'flat response' hearing aid. The probe tube at the bottom of each earmold measures the dB in SPL at the eardrum and displays the results. Now, each modification is visible.

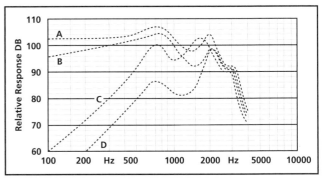

Fig. 16-8
Frequency Response

A. Represents a solid mold in the ear canal.

B. Represents shortening the mold, which reduces the overall output a few dB up to about 2000 Hz.

C. Represents a small vent to the outside air, a parallel vent. Notice what happens to the lower frequencies. While they 'bleed off', sounds become boosted above 1000 Hz. Now the opening in the mold allows some ear canal resonance.

D. Represents an open tube fitting, with the skeleton of the mold holding the tube in place. The ear perceives only extremely high frequency emphasis. Ear canal resonance functions normally, with a 'boost' from amplification.

A systematic relationship exists between the amount of earmold material removed from the ear canal, the size of the parallel vent and the amount of filtering in the lower frequencies.

Sound takes the easy way out. It is easier to escape through the air vent than to force the eardrum to vibrate.

Remember, too, that low frequencies give us the power or loudness of speech. Each successive change in the above modifications **does reduce the lower frequencies, making the remaining sounds appear quieter.** UCL changes as well, but it usually rises approximately 5 dB when the mold is vented to the outside air. The overall sound is quieter when the lows are not present.

The shape of the audiogram does not always indicate the need for a particular response slope. Use of the audiogram only may be misleading when applied to hearing instrument needs or fittings. The choice of earmold and related modifications can drastically alter any response slope.

The shape of the audiogram is a good guide to the selection of earmolds, along with the knowledge of how the slope is altered. The Earmolds lesson covers this in more detail.

Frequency Response: If we want to 'tilt' the frequency response, first we must be able to read a frequency response graph.

Hearing instrument analyzers measure frequency response. A frequency response curve involves introducing a 60 dB SPL tone at each frequency and recording how much the hearing instrument amplifies at several discrete frequencies, then printing a graph of the frequency response.

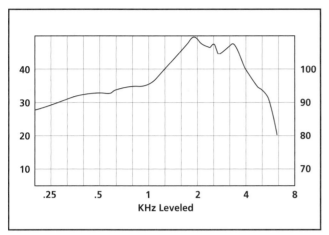

Fig. 16-9
Gain Curve

Gain: If we want to know the gain of the hearing instrument, we subtract the input (60 dB), and the identical curve becomes a **gain curve.** The readings on the left hand side are 60 dB less, expressing gain instead of frequency response.

Tilting the Frequency Response: Tilting or filtering the frequency response can be accomplished in several ways. You have already seen how an outside vent in the earmold tilts the response drastically.

We can describe tilting the frequency response as gain per octave, for instance, a 6 dB per octave rise. The frequency response shows 6 dB more at 1000 Hz than at 500 Hz, and another 6 dB at 2000 Hz. Limits of hearing instrument circuits do not do the high frequency area justice, so base the dB/octave on either 500 Hz or 1000 Hz.

Tilting the frequency response can also use a matrix, for instance l08/30/15. The first number is the output of the hearing instrument, corresponding to UCL, the second number represents the peak gain of the instrument, and the last number relates to the rise in the frequency response between 500 Hz and the first peak on the frequency response graph. Each time you 'tilt' the frequency response from 'flat' response, the sound becomes quieter. More volume is required to keep the comfortable level.

Hearing instruments have tone controls, or frequency response potentiometers (pots) that will also accomplish this task. Some models are designed to give a wide, flat response, while others use high frequency emphasis. You can use a combination of a filtered response, venting and tone controls.

Anyone with hearing loss is a candidate for hearing instrument use. Hearing loss is a **handicap.** Audiometric thresholds and SRT are poor indicators of the degree of handicap a patient experiences.

Successful Fitting: No one wears hearing instruments for prestige, status symbols, or cosmetic appeal. Deal with the handicap. **The determining factors, need and desire on the patient's part, create the motivation necessary for successful hearing instrument use.**

The **general attitude of the patient** affects their motivation. For some people, a borderline loss is devastating. Their livelihood depends on hearing and understanding low intensity speech sounds. Others, living or working in less critical listening situations, approach 40 - 50 dB thresholds before detecting hearing loss.

Age restricts both handling and use. The patient is slower to respond. They may have dexterity problems. They may find difficulty coping with noisy or chaotic situations.

At the other end of the age scale, fitting children requires close co-operation with an Otologist and Clinical Audiologist.

Cosmetic appeal is important. Regardless of age, the patient wants an inconspicuous hearing instrument. Patients in their 80's and 90's question the visibility of a hearing instrument, and respond to the reaction of others.

The client accepts the hearing instrument only if it fulfills their cosmetic and personal wishes. These wishes are as important as any performance considerations.

Use Time: Successful hearing instrument users do not wear their hearing instrument all the time. **Use time** is not a basis for a successful fitting. Assessing use time is less important than fulfilling their hearing need.

Degree of Loss: The **degree of loss** often determines both satisfaction with hearing instrument and use time.

Mild loss is slight for some and significant for others. Sustained attention is difficult.

People with **moderate losses** hear someone close without difficulty. Their speech often shows articulation omissions, substitutions and distortions. They benefit from a hearing instrument.

Moderately Severe loss patients understand loud conversational speech, but have difficulty in groups or noise. They have enough hearing to use auditory feedback to learn or maintain speech, and gain excellent benefit from a hearing instrument.

Patients with **severe losses** hear loud sounds or a voice close to the ear. They even identify environmental noises or vowels, but miss consonants. A hearing instrument lets them function for ordinary purposes.

Profound losses do not rely on hearing for communication. The hearing instrument cannot compensate for the hearing impairment. A hearing instrument maintains contact with the environment and allows them an awareness of what is going on around them, using auditory clues.

Slope of Loss: The **slope of loss** also plays a part in a successful fitting.

Most favorable is the flat, gradually rising or falling loss. Less favorable is steep falling, deep saucer shape, or irregular dips and peaks in audiometric thresholds. Least favorable is a sharp drop at any lower frequency, islands of hearing only, or remnants of hearing in the low frequencies.

Discrimination Scores: Discrimination scores also offer some general rules.

90%   Good results with a hearing instrument.

70 - 90%   Hearing instruments offer a mild difference.

50 - 70%   Notices a substantial difference.

50% or less   Finds amplification not entirely successful.

METHODS of HEARING INSTRUMENT SELECTION

We know that a properly fitted hearing instrument does not alter or improve any condition or characteristic of a pathological ear. We can only make sound louder in a controlled manner, improving the patient's ability to function and communicate.

Just as there are different ways of looking at hearing loss, there are differing methods on how to achieve functional acuity, based on threshold, MCL, UCL, or speech spectra.

Each method must amplify sound within a comfortable range, and improve hearing acuity or it is rejected by the patient. The calculation of amplified sound for the patient to use at their comfortable level is **use gain, operating gain, functional gain, or estimated insertion gain.** The hearing instrument also requires **reserve gain** so the patient can adjust the volume as required.

Any method describing gain at each frequency is a **Prescriptive Method.** Any method comparing one product, slope, frequency, output or other measurement with another is a **Comparative Method.**

The International Hearing Society does not endorse any particular fitting method. We encourage our members to be familiar with the advantages and the disadvantages of a large number of fitting procedures. From this knowledge, you find procedures that seem most feasible and most objective for fitting hearing instruments.

COMPARATIVE METHODS

Pressure Measuring Instruments (PMI's): One approach to hearing instrument selection explores 'tilting' the response curve using a PMI - Pressure Measuring Instrument, to increase or decrease specific frequencies in the speech range until the response is no longer flat.

We can evaluate the patient in different listening conditions, compare discrimination scores and verify our controlled settings with left, right or binaural amplification.

PMI's go by several other names, SPL Audiometer, Master Hearing Instrument, Hearing instrument Simulator, Hearing instrument Comparator, Auricon, etc. The circuitry in PMI's closely approximates the circuitry in hearing instruments. Your patient experiences

listening with amplification prior to being fitted with a hearing instrument, and hears with either ear or both ears together in a variety of listening situations. The patient becomes an active participant in the decision making process.

You can demonstrate quality hearing in real life situations, with either ear alone, or both ears together. No amount of discussion can replace this experience for either of you.

Carhart Procedure: This procedure emphasizes speech discrimination scores in quiet and in noise, and aided SRT and tolerance thresholds, using several different models of hearing instruments for comparison.

Comparison is often the best alternative in severe to profound losses, where the patient functions in abnormal critical band widths and can detect qualities that escape your measurements, or in bone conduction fittings.

Mirroring the Audiogram: This concept involves providing enough gain at each frequency to correct the pure tone sensitivity to normal, or 0 dB. Although the idea appears obvious to the uninformed, impaired ears do not respond to sound in the same way as normal ears. It is virtually impossible to fit the gain required in the higher frequencies without exceeding UCL. This concept also does not take into account the differences between SPL in the hearing instrument and HL on the audiogram, where dB values are not the same, or any effects of earmold acoustics.

Even with all these drawbacks, we tend to 'assume' some of this concept from the slope of the audiogram in the fitting of hearing instruments. We certainly use the audiogram for the selection of molds.

Equal Loudness Contours: Find MCL for a 1000 Hz tone, then find the intensity required to match this loudness at specific frequencies. The frequency response mirrors the difference between the patient's equal loudness contour and the auditory threshold.

Although this method is very time consuming, speech discrimination scores are reported to be much better than when using relative gain or shaping the frequency response. Difficult-to-test subjects find loudness matching too sophisticated a task.

Bisection Procedure: The bisection procedure finds the midpoint of the dynamic range between 1000 Hz and 4000 Hz, using the difference between UCL - SRT. A downward slope of 8 - 10 dB per octave below 1000 Hz avoids any low frequency masking effects.

Otometry: A majority of the principles of John Victoreen and Otometry are in use today in many forms.

Otometry measures threshold, most comfortable loudness, and UCL at each frequency, using a damped wave train in SPL instead of pure tones. A damped wave train tone burst has a specified decay rate. The gain characteristics of the hearing instrument raise average amplified spectra of speech to MCL for normal ears.

PRESCRIPTIVE METHODS

Prescriptive methods divide, add or multiply factors, based on audiometric HL at each frequency. Some methods also use correction factors to reduce the gain in the lower frequencies and avoid the upward spread of masking, or as compensation for other fitting choices. The gain necessary to reach comfort level at each frequency is use gain. Allowance is made for reserve gain.

The Half Gain Formula: This formula gives a practical general guideline, suggesting the gain requirement to reach MCL through the hearing instrument is approximately one-half the pure tone ANSI thresholds. Add 10 - 15 dB reserve gain, so the patient wears the hearing instrument less than full volume.

Libby Procedure: One-third HTL at each frequency, minus 5 dB at 250 Hz and 3 dB at 500 Hz.

Lybarger Method: One-third HTL at 500 Hz, one-half HTL at 1000 - 4000 Hz.

Skinner Procedure for Ski-Slope Losses: Select the frequency-gain characteristic of the instrument so amplified conversational speech falls in the middle of the dynamic range. High frequency emphasis does not exceed 15 dB for balance between 500 Hz - 1000 Hz, and 2000 Hz - 4000 Hz presentation levels.

FORMULAS USING INSERTION GAIN

1/3, 1/2, 2/3 GAIN

Frequency (Hz)	HTL (dB)	Factor (÷) 1/3	1/2	2/3	Correction	Estimated Insertion Gain
250		3	2	1.5	-5	
500		3	2	1.5	-3	
1000		3	2	1.5	0	
2000		3	2	1.5	0	
3000		3	2	1.5	0	
4000		3	2	1.5	0	
6000		3	2	1.5	-5	

POGO

Frequency (Hz)	HTL (dB)	Factor (÷)	Correction	Estimated Insertion Gain
250		2	-10	
500		2	-3	
1000		2	0	
2000		2	0	
3000		2	0	
4000		2	0	

BERGER

Frequency (Hz)	HTL (dB)	Factor (÷)	Estimated Insertion Gain
500		2	
1000		1.6	
2000		1.5	
3000		1.7	
4000		2	
* 6000		2	

* See correction factors

N.A.L.

Frequency (Hz)	X + 0.31 (HTL)*	Correction (dB)	Estimated Insertion Gain
250	X + 0.31 ( )	-17	
500	X + 0.31 ( )	-8	
750	X + 0.31 ( )	-3	
1000	X + 0.31 ( )	+1	
1500	X + 0.31 ( )	+1	
2000	X + 0.31 ( )	-1	
3000	X + 0.31 ( )	-2	
4000	X + 0.31 ( )	-2	
6000	X + 0.31 ( )	-2	

* X = 0.05 (HTL @ 500 Hz) +
(HTL @ 1000 Hz) +
(HTL @ 2000 Hz)

500 Hz _____

1000 Hz _____

+ 2000 Hz _____

Total _____

X 0.05 _____

X = _____

Fig. 17-1

Data on severely impaired individuals found the preferred gain setting about +7 dB above hearing threshold levels. On the basis of this data, the Pogo (Prescription of Gain and Output) formula, was modified for hearing losses greater than 65 dB.

Pogo II: For Hearing Loss greater than 65 dB. Correction factors remain 10 dB less at 250 Hz and 5 dB less at 500 Hz.

Insertion Gain = half the hearing level + half the hearing level minus 65. For example, a threshold of 80 dB at 2000 Hz is $80 \div 2 = 40 + (80 - 65 \div 2 = 7.5) = 47.5$ dB gain.

Correction Factors: Correction factors in the Berger Procedure are as follows:

If microphone placement is a behind the ear fitting, add 2 dB at 2000 Hz and 3 dB at 3000 Hz for loss of Pinna effect.

When using a body-worn instrument, reduce gain at 500 Hz, and add at 2000 Hz to overcome body baffle effect.

Subtract 3 dB for a binaural fitting.

Use 1/5 of the air-bone gap added to operating gain for a conductive component.

All procedures are guidelines based on averages, and some adjustments may be necessary for individual requirements.

Prescriptive calculations are not the exact replica of the gain curve of the hearing instrument. The calculations are the basis for comparison to hearing instrument specification sheets. Use of these calculations includes earmolds and modifications in combination with a hearing instrument frequency response, discussed in the chapter on Hearing instruments.

Uncomfortable Loudness Levels: Uncomfortable loudness levels, regardless of the method of measurement, must be in SPL to fit a hearing instrument.

HL narrow band UCL's convert at each frequency.

HL speech UCL thresholds convert using ANSI Standards of 20 dB.

PMI tolerance thresholds are SPL.

Prescription formulas also determine the UCL limits of a hearing instrument. When discussing these limits, **output, MPO (Maximum Power Output), and SSPL (Saturation Sound Pressure Level) become the technical terms.** We can use our pre-measured calculations, or convert UCL to a Prescription Formula in SSPL.

Pogo: HL UCL at $\underline{500 \text{ Hz} + 1000 \text{ Hz} + 2000 \text{ Hz}}$ + 4 dB

3

The 4 dB is a SPL conversion factor, and is slightly lower than converting each HL frequency.

Berger Procedure: Berger has a different way of looking at UCL. A hearing instrument does not need to exactly match UCL, must not exceed UCL, and should amplify louder speech sounds without distortion.

Berger recommends measuring 500, 1000, 2000 and 4000 Hz with pulsed pure tones, then convert HL to SPL. These levels become **Maximum Permissable SSPL.**

The level where loud speech sounds are amplified without distortion is the **Minimum Desirable SSPL. Using the** Berger calculated insertion gain at each frequency, add

      75 dB at 500 Hz

      75 dB at 1000 Hz

      72 dB at 2000 Hz

      70 dB at 4000 Hz to obtain the Minimum Desirable SSPL at each frequency.

You can limit the hearing instrument output anywhere between minimum and maximum SSPL. Whenever the minimum exceeds maximum, use the lowest (maximum) amount.

TYPES of FITTINGS

Monaural: A **monaural fitting** uses one hearing instrument on either the left or the right ear.

> **Head Shadow Effect:** The head blocks sound arriving from the unamplified side, causing high frequency attenuation. Low frequency sounds travel around the head easier than high frequency sounds. Signal-to-noise ratios between the two ears vary as much as 13 dB because of the head shadow effect.

> **Auditory Deprivation:** Auditory deprivation occurs with prolonged use of amplification to one ear. The ear without amplification loses its ability to discriminate, with measurable differences in a 4 to 5 year period, while the aided ear discrimination scores remain stable over time.

Binaural: A **binaural fitting** requires the use of two hearing instruments, one on each ear. Binaural ear-level instruments restore a semblance of normal binaural auditory functioning, but two body-worn instruments do not.

Some patients do have a bias, either for or against, binaural fittings. Because our responsibility is to the patient, our attitudes with regard to binaural fittings are both important and influential. We do not have the right to allow the patient to think a monaural fitting is acceptable unless there is a contra-indication to binaural from our test results.

Contra-indications to Binaural Fitting

1. Degradation effect - When binaural discrimination scores are poorer than with the better ear alone.

2. Poor Binaural Fusion - audiometric thresholds are greatly asymmetrical and often longstanding.

3. Dynamic Range - one ear has a small dynamic range.

4. Diplacusis - a patient who perceives a different pitch on each ear is a poor binaural candidate.

5. UCL very low in one ear. These patients also have small dynamic range.

6. Patients with a psychological feeling of being closed-off or plugged or confined with both ears occluded.

7. Physical factors such as multiple disabilities or motor skills dysfunction.

Bilateral: A **bilateral fitting (Y-cord)** uses one body-worn hearing instrument with a 'Y' shaped cord and a receiver and earmold in each ear. Thresholds must be symmetrical.

BiCros: A **BiCros fitting** uses one complete hearing instrument on the better ear and a second microphone on the non-functional ear.

Cros: Use a **Cros fitting** for a person with unilateral loss or a non-functional ear, and normal hearing on the better ear.

Bone Conduction: Bone conduction fittings are useful for bilateral atresia, chronic draining ears, or massive conductive components with sensorineural involvement.

Potentially Unaidable Ears

1. Profound sensorineural loss where maximum amplification cannot reach the patient's thresholds.

2. Severe or profound mixed losses, like atresia.

3. An abnormally small dynamic range, i.e., 5 dB.

4. Abnormally low UCL's.

5. Very poor discrimination that degrades the better ear.

6. Ear under medical treatment.

7. Otolaryngologist recommends amplification be avoided.

INTERNATIONAL
INSTITUTE
FOR
HEARING
INSTRUMENTS
STUDIES

DISTANCE LEARNING
for Professionals in
HEARING HEALTH SCIENCES

RATIONALE FOR CIC FITTINGS

LESSON 18

The first commercially available deep canal hearing instrument or Completely-in-the-Canal hearing aid (CIC) was introduced to the European market in 1991 and five years later made up 12% of all hearing aids sold in the United States. During the time that CICs have been available for fitting, manufacturers, hearing instrument practitioners and consumers have gained considerable knowledge regarding this small and popular form of amplification. CIC fittings provide patients with unique advantages while compelling the hearing instrument practitioner to alter their fitting procedures and validation methods slightly.

ADVANTAGES OF CIC FITTINGS

Reduction of the Occlusion Effect

When a person speaks or moves their jaw, the ear canal walls within the cartilaginous portion of the ear canal change shape, setting air particles in motion within the ear canal. Without a hearing aid in the ear, the air particles are channeled out of the canal. With an aid in place they are forced to flow inward, resulting in the perception of the patient's own voice being louder, scratchy and unpleasant. This effect has been termed the Occlusion Effect and due to the increase in bone-conducted sound for frequencies below 2000 Hz when the external ear or ear canal is covered. It has long been believed that when an earplug is inserted more deeply into the inner bony one-third of the external ear canal, it reduces the occlusion effect, providing an alternative to the traditional form of occlusion effect reduction, which is increased venting. The amount of occlusion effect reduction varies by patient and by CIC, but overall, patient's voices should be rendered more natural with CIC fittings.

Increase in High Frequency Emphasis

The microphone, by definition of the aid being a CIC, must fit down into the ear canal. This deeper placed microphone disrupts the ear's own natural resonance less than other forms of amplification, allowing for a greater retention of the ear's ability to transmit sounds between 2000-4000 Hz more efficiently. Both the primary resonance at around 2700 Hz can be preserved to some degree as with the secondary resonate peak of 4000-5000 Hz. This allows for increased high frequency amplification without placing additional demands upon the hearing aid circuit. The following figure demonstrates, via real-ear insertion gain, the increased high frequency gain associated with CICs when compared to other forms of amplication.

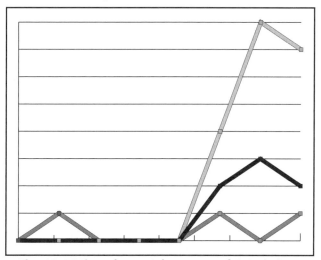

Fig. 18-1 Microphone Advantage of CIC Fittings

Gain Reduction

As CICs fit closer to the tympanic membrane and the residual cavity between the tip of the ear canal and the eardrum is smaller, less gain is required from the hearing aid to provide the same amount of amplification to the patient. While this seems impossible, it is similar to placing the same radio at the same volume into a very small room, such as a closet versus a very large room such as an auditorium. The radio will sound louder in the closet than in the auditorium even though the sound is equally loud. Since a prescribed amount of amplification is required based upon the hearing loss, if the cavity is smaller, the hearing aid can provide less gain to sound equally loud. This allows for greater degrees of hearing loss to be fit with the same gain circuits and for patients to use less gain with their instruments which has advantages in reducing feedback and increasing battery life.

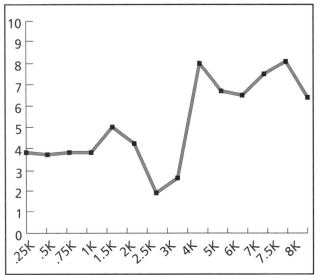

Fig. 18-2 Averaged Real-Ear Insertion Gain Difference by Frequency with CIC's-vs-ITE Fittings

Reduction in Feedback

Typically, CICs provide very small pressure equalization venting or no venting at all, with venting one of the major sources of chronic feedback with hearing aids. In addition, as has been mentioned, less gain is required for CIC fittings. Finally, CIC fittings are usually more tightly fitting than other forms of amplification. These three variables provide for a reduction in feedback for patients.

Undistorted Output

A benefit of using less gain is the ability to have an increase in output that is distortion free or increased headroom. Headroom describes the condition that occurs when the input plus the gain of the hearing aid does not exceed the SSPL90 of the hearing aid. Once the SSPL90 of the hearing aid is exceeded, the hearing aid is said to be in saturation and is distorting. If we suppose that a patient is in an environment which is 70 dB SPL, and the CIC hearing aid that the patient is wearing only requires 15 dB gain,

the total output equals 85 dB which is underneath the SSPL90 value associated with distortion. However, should the same patient require the use of another style of hearing aid with 30 dB of amplification to meet their gain requirements, the 30 dB SPL added to the 70 dB SPL environmental condition, will force their hearing aid into saturation, as the output of 100 dB SPL would exceed the upper level of their hearing aid.

	CIC	Other
Gain	15	30
Input	70	70
Total Output:	85	100

Miscellaneous Advantages

Due to the deeper microphone placement, CICs have been found to have a decrease in Wind Noise. While wind noise was found to be reduced by 7 dB SPL when compared to ITE fittings for wind coming from all directions, when the wind was coming from directly ahead, the CIC offered 23 dB less wind noise.

Telephone Use is facilitated when using CICs due to the reduction of feedback with a deeper microphone placement. Additionally, use of Stethoscopes and Headsets are facilitated for the same reason.

Some researchers have reported an increase in Intelligibility in Noise with CICs that is presumably due to creating a large real ear occluded response-or creating the maximum "earplug" effect with the hearing aid in but not turned on, which attenuates the response of the hearing aid over a wide range of frequencies. This attenuation lessens the level of background noise, improving signal to noise ratio. Essentially, the hearing aid acts as an earplug and then only those frequencies that are required for speech are amplified.

Miscellaneous Disadvantages

It would not be fitting to list advantages of CIC fittings without describing disadvantages as well. Fortunately, the advantages outweigh the disadvantages but several disadvantages still remain:

While feedback reduction was listed as an advantage, it must be listed as a disadvantage as well. Chronic Feedback due to mandibular joint movement plagues some patients. Manufacturers have various suggestions for reducing this phenomenon but even after following the manufacture guidelines, some patients are not successfully fit or are fit in the office, but the hearing aid works itself out of the ear when chewing or talking. Canal locks, open jaw impressions or built up rings/spirals of soft/hard materials are but a few of the suggestions manufacturers have for reducing this problem.

Due to size limitations, the patient's ability to manipulate the hearing aid is severely limited. Many CICs are fit without volume controls and without dispenser or patient controls. This lack of fitting flexibility has been reduced with the introduction of programmable CICs but many CICs still have less fitting flexibility than their larger counterparts.

Cost is also a current limitation. CICs have a higher percentage of returns and are more difficult for manufacturers to produce so costs remain higher for these smaller instruments.

FITTING PROCEDURE ALTERATION

The following are general suggestions for alteration of traditional fitting procedure. It should be noted that each manufacture has unique suggestions for alteration and the manufacturer of choice should be contacted to insure that their procedures are carried out when taking impressions, ordering a circuit or prescribing a material.

Impression Techniques

While a satisfactory impression is critical for all hearing aid orders, with CICs the impression process becomes even more critical. An adequately long ear impression is imperative, at least 2 mm beyond the second bend is mandatory to insure appropriate sound direction and canal direction.

Silicon impression material is strongly recommended for CIC impressions, as it is less likely to stretch when being removed from the ear canal. Medium viscosity materials are recommended both for patient comfort and the degree that they remain true to the ear canal shape.

Special earblocks are recommended. This can vary from oiled cotton blocks which take up less room in the ear canal than foam blocks while providing a stable barrier to the impression material, to vented blocks which allow for air equalization, to special blocks provided by the manufacturer.

The mandible plays a unique role with CIC fittings and consequently, due to the different shaped impressions obtained from different jaw positions, some manufacturers recommend taking an open jaw impression, while others recommend having the patient remain quiet or chewing/talking while taking an impression of the patient's ear.

Circuit Selection

The frequency response of the CIC will vary from that of other forms of amplification for a variety of reasons. Using a prescriptive formula for gain that has not been altered for CIC fittings will result in the CIC being too strong or loud. CIC corrections must be used to insure that the gain expected in the ear canal is obtained. As the hearing aid is being placed into a cavity much smaller than the ANSI 2-cc coupler typically used for verification, the gain values obtained from the manufacturer will appear weaker than expected. When making measurements in the office, either a smaller CIC coupler must be used to more adequately predict the gain in the ear canal or correction factors should be employed.

The slope of the CIC hearing aid must often be flatter for patients than would be anticipated, providing an increase in low frequency amplification. This is particularly true if the patient has normal low frequency hearing acuity. The small pinhole vent and tight fit of CICs does not allow for low frequency transfer of sound information, as is the case for other types of amplification. Without this low frequency information, the patient will report that they do not hear as well with their hearing aid as without it, and when tested the patients will demonstrate a low frequency hearing loss with the hearing aid in. The hearing aid is, essentially, acting as an earplug. By increasing the low frequency emphasis of the circuit, his problem is eliminated.

As has been previously mentioned, the deep microphone placement of a CIC hearing aid allows for a natural retention of high frequency emphasis at 2700-4000 Hz. This retention must be taken into consideration when prescribing the amount of high frequency gain required to avoid over amplification and a shrill, harsh sound quality. A reduction in high frequency gain provided by the instrument will allow for fitting criteria to be met.

With instruments that do not have volume controls that allow patients to limit amplification upon demand, increased attention must be placed on circuits that allow for automatic gain reduction in loud environments. Many such circuits allow for patients to comfortably wear their hearing aids without being dependent upon a volume control.

Manufacturing Methods

Many CIC hearing aids are produced using different shell materials and designs than their larger counterparts. These shell materials, such as ultraviolet shells, often require additional skills for modification as well as other types of materials/equipment for in office patching, building up or buffing. Materials and methods vary from manufacturer to manufacturer but it is imperative that the materials used for modification be compatible with the manufacturer being used for hearing aid production.

VALIDATION METHODS

Real Ear Measurement

With traditional real measurement, it is recommended that the probe be placed at least 4 mm beyond the tip of the hearing aid in order to avoid transitional field or evanescent wave artifacts in the higher frequency range. In addition, it is recommended that the tip of the probe be placed within 5 mm of the eardrum to avoid standing waves. Finally, due to the low frequency transfer of energy through the acoustic vent, it is never recommended that the probe be inserted through the vent.

With CIC fittings, only the middle statement of the above three statements remains true. The probe should be within 5 mm of the eardrum to avoid standing waves but provided the tip extends beyond the end of the ear canal of the CIC, no appreciable difference in frequency response will be obtained.

As feedback with CIC fittings with a probe in place often creates problems with real ear measurements; the probe can be inserted through the vent. The vent of a CIC does not allow for significant acoustic transfer of low frequency information so placing the probe through the vent or along side the aid will provide virtually the same information.

Functional Gain Under Headphones

Functional gain allows us to compare unaided results with aided results, and are usually obtained using sound field stimulation. Sound field stimulation has distinct disadvantages due to the test-retest reliability with patient head movement and the inability to test each ear independently. With CIC fittings, just as most patients are able to use the telephone, a stethoscope or headset, functional gain measurements can be obtained under headphones.

The advantage of this form of functional gain testing is that it has less test-retest variability and allows for each ear to be assessed independently. In addition, it is simple for the patient to understand and appreciate the improvement between unaided and aided thresholds. An audiogram, such as the one in Figure 18-3 could easily demonstrate the improvement in threshold via this method. However, functional gain is more time consuming and less comprehensive than real-ear measure**ment.**

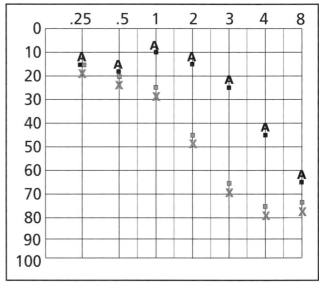

Fig. 18-3 Functional Gain via Headphones (A=Aided Responses / X=Unaided Responses)

HEARING INSTRUMENTS / DIGITAL TECHNOLOGY

LESSON 19

Digital technology is not new to hearing instruments. It was used in commercially available hearing instruments as early as the mid 1980's, with the Zeta Noise Blocker filter, and flourished with the introduction of digitally programmable hearing instruments in the late 1980's.

A "true" digital processing hearing instrument was created in 1983 by Audiotone, but it was never produced commercially. The first commercially available digital processing hearing instrument was the Phoenix, manufactured by Nicollet. Introduced in 1988, the Phoenix was a BTE instrument that featured user controllable multiple-memory selection and noise reduction, and processing to change the frequency response, gain, and SSPL90 of the hearing instrument. It also, however, included less desirable features such as: a body-worn electronic processor/battery pack and cable attachment to each instrument, very poor battery life, and expensive proprietary hardware for programming. Needless to say, it was not a commercial success.

Advancements in VLSI (Very Large Scale Integration) and CMOS (Complimentary Metal Oxide Semi-Conductor) technology has fostered the development of extremely small microprocessors that can house numerous components in a small area and operate on low power and voltage. This has helped to facilitate the introduction of "true" digital processing hearing instruments that can be packaged in smaller sizes and yield effective performance with the nominal 1.3V batteries used in hearing instruments.

ANALOG VS. DIGITAL

The term "analog", which is derived from the word "analogous", refers to data in the form of continuously changing physical quantities. One of the most common analog signals is the sine wave. The molecules of air move back and forth in a smooth and continuous motion. In an analog electronic system, the voltage level increases and decreases smoothly and continuously.

Digital, on the other hand, refers to data in the form of discrete units. As the name implies, digital devices process information that is in a numerical format. Continuity is replaced by discreteness and a highly constrained, finite set of symbols. In a digital system, numbers are used to describe the size of the signal at certain points in time. As the voltage increases, the number increases in predefined increments or steps.

The difference between analog and digital can be easily seen through the operation of analog and digital clocks. The second hand of an analog clock continuously sweeps along, allowing us to tell if it is 5, 5 1/2 , or 5 3/4, minutes after 10 o'clock. A digital clock, however, will be limited by the smallest increment used. If the smallest increment used is minutes, then we will only be able to tell if it is 5 or 6 minutes after 10 o'clock. The accuracy of the system is limited (or enhanced) by the smallest increment used.

WHY DIGITAL PROCESSING

Today's analog circuitry is capable of performing sophisticated signal processing but there is a limit to the amount and variety of the processing that can be accomplished in the small sizes required for hearing instruments. Digital signals can be manipulated with greater precision and reliability, and less additive noise, compared to analog processing. Potential advantages of digital sound processing are: Lower noise and higher fidelity (internal noise should be limited only by the quality of the microphone and the receiver), extensive processing capability (very specialized functions are possible), and the capability to load a variety of processing schemes into one hearing instrument via software (DSP systems having this capability are termed Open Platform).

As research reveals more effective ways of processing sound for the hearing impaired and as the complexity of the desired processing increases, digital signal processing will be required to implement these processing schemes effectively. While DSP may provide enhancements to the kinds of processing that can be performed by analog hearing instruments, the real power of DSP lies in the ability to perform processing functions that analog hearing instruments cannot do.

ANALOG HEARING INSTRUMENTS

Any hearing instrument that is not a "true" or "fully" digital hearing instrument, is an analog hearing instrument. Inside the analog hearing instrument, voltages are amplified and filtered. At any point in the process, if you examined the voltages inside the hearing instrument with an oscilloscope, you would find a continuously varying waveform. Digital components can, however, be added to create more versatile systems.

HYBRID ANALOG-DIGITAL HEARING INSTRUMENTS

A hybrid analog-digital hearing instrument is one that contains a digital computer chip to control some aspect of how sound is amplified. While the hearing instrument remains an analog system (the signal is always in analog

form), digital components are used to control the filtering or compression characteristics. Since digital technology is used in some fashion with an analog hearing instrument, the term "hybrid" can be applied, because it indicates a merging of two types of technologies. (This should not be confused, however, with the term "hybrid" as it refers to a method of manufacturing electronic components).

One example of an analog hearing instrument incorporating a digital chip for filtering was the Zeta Noise Blocker (ZNB). The Zeta Noise Blocker was a digital chip implemented with ITE analog hearing instruments for noise-reduction, in the mid 1980's. The ZNB attempted to separate speech from noise in several frequency bands using temporal differences between speech and quasi-steady state noise. The ZNB was not successful because it produced too-noticeable changes in the frequency response from only small changes in the listening environment.

DIGITALLY PROGRAMMABLE HEARING INSTRUMENTS

The digitally programmable hearing instrument, also referred to as digitally controlled analog (DCA), is also a hybrid because there is a digital component inside the hearing instrument. But unlike the Zeta Noise Blocker, whose purpose was to perform filtering, the digital components are present for the purpose of programming the parameters of the hearing instrument. The frequency response, gain, MPO, and compression parameters are

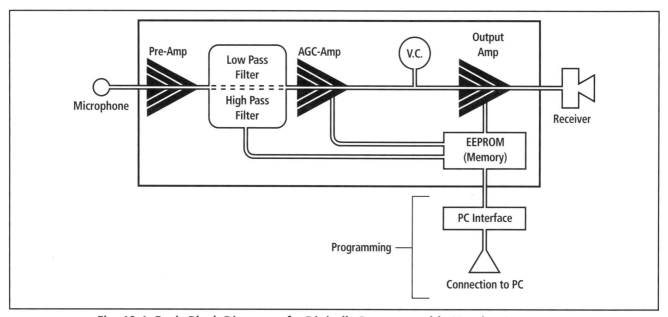

Fig. 19-1 Basic Block Diagram of a Digitally Programmable Hearing Instrument

set by attaching the hearing instrument to a computer or other digital device as opposed to using trimpots. This type of system consists of two primary components; the hearing instrument which contains a memory chip where the selected settings are stored, and the programming device which is used by the fitter for adjusting the settings. Figure 19-1 shows a basic block diagram of a digitally programmable hearing instrument.

Digitally programmable hearing instruments, first introduced in the late 1980's have capabilities that result in increased flexibility and more precise fittings. Parameters such as gain, MPO, and frequency response can be selected and adjusted for the wearer while hc/she is wearing the hearing instrument. And, if different settings are required to account for subjective preferences or hearing loss changes, reprogramming to these settings can usually be accomplished without needing to return the instrument to the manufacturer. Additionally, advanced signal processing such as multiple-channel compression, and the use of wearer accessible multiple memories (different parameter settings for different listening environments), can be implemented most effectively with digitally programmable hearing instruments.

Programmable hearing instruments can be classified according to their features. One such classification scheme places hearing instruments into four classes, based upon the number of channels and memories. These classes are:

Class 1: Single Channel/Single Memory;

Class 2: Single Channel/Multiple Memory;

Class 3: Multiple Channel/Single Memory;

Class 4: Multiple Channel/Multiple Memory.

This classification system is depicted in Figure 19-2.

	Single Channel = 1	Multiple Channel > 1
Single Memory = 1	CLASS 1	CLASS 3
Multiple Memory > 1	CLASS 2	CLASS 4

Fig. 19-2 Programmable Hearing Insruments classified by number of memories and channels

DESCRIPTION OF MEMORY

As previously mentioned, a digital memory is used to store the hearing instrument parameter settings. There are different types of digital storage mechanisms available in semiconductor memory. These consist of RAM (Random Access Memory), PROM (Programmable Read-Only Memory), EPROM (Erasable Programmable Read-Only Memory), and EEPROM (Electrically Erasable Programmable Read-Only Memory). RAM can have data written to and read from it in any random order, but requires a second backup voltage supply to store the programmed parameters. Thus, if there isn't a backup voltage supply (battery), when the hearing instrument is turned off or the battery is changed, the instructions are lost and have to be reloaded again from the programmer.

PROM allows the parameters to be stored only once, requiring a physical change in the PROM chip to change hearing instrument performance. EPROM allows the programmed parameters to be changed after subjecting the digital memory to an ultraviolet light in order to erase it. EEPROM can have data written into it, or read from it, and may also have new data rewritten and stored. EEPROM allows the stored parameters to be changed using a programming instrument.

NOAH

Digitally programmable hearing instruments using different technologies and different programming devices were introduced from a number of manufacturers. Dispensers who wanted to dispense multiple brands of programmable hearing instruments found it necessary to invest in, store, maintain, and learn to use multiple programmable fitting systems. In order to find an alternative to this often costly and inconvenient process, a group of hearing instrument manufacturers, audiological test equipment firms, and office management software companies worked together to develop an integrated hearing care software system, called NOAH. NOAH uses a common software platform and central database to integrate hearing instrument fitting systems, test equipment, and office management software systems. NOAH integrates client records, audiological data, client journals, and the dedicated fitting and measurement modules from various companies. It provides a common software platform for multiple brands of programmable hearing instruments, allowing the dispenser to use a personal computer (PC) to fit a variety of hearing instruments within one system.

DIGITAL SIGNAL PROCESSING HEARING INSTRUMENTS (OVERVIEW)

Digital signal processing refers to the process of breaking up a signal into discrete sets of binary numbers that represent the signal, performing various mathematical operations on those numbers, and then converting the result back into a real-world, analog signal.

There are three basic stages of a digital system:

- analog-to-digital conversion
- processing algorithm
- digital-to-analog conversion

In a hearing instrument, the analog-to-digital conversion takes an analog signal from the microphone and breaks it into a series of numbers. Each number in the series represents the signal at a specific time. These numbers are then manipulated by the processing algorithm.

A processing algorithm is a defined set of mathematical steps involving multiplication, addition, and subtraction. These relatively simple operations are combined in complex sequences to accomplish filtering, amplification, attenuation, and other processing steps, which are stored as a computer program. A signal processor, then, is a highly optimized microprocessor that performs these program steps thousands of times a second, allowing for greater control of the signal than is available with an analog system.

The remaining stage is the digital-to-analog conversion. Here, the results of the processing algorithm, which is still a series of numbers, is converted back into an analog real-world signal. In hearing instruments, the converted signal is produced by the hearing instrument receiver.

BINARY NUMBERS

A binary number is a number consisting of the digits 0 and 1. With a binary code, when a 0 is placed on the end of the number string, the value of the number is doubled. In contrast, the addition of a 0 at the end of a decimal system number indicates a multiplication of 10. A simple binary progression contrasted to the more familiar decimal code is shown in Figure 19-3.

The number of code combinations increase significantly each time the amount of numbers, referred to as bits, is doubled. A string of 4 bits can be formed into 16 possible states or permutations, 8 bits can be formed into

256 possible states, and a 16 bit binary number has 65,536 possible states. Thus, there is a significant relationship between the number of bits and increased complexity of signal representation.

Decimal System		Binary Code
0		0
1		1
2		10
3		11
4		100
5		101
6		110
7		111
8		1000
9		1001
10		1010
16		10000
32		100000
64		1000000
128		10000000

With permission from Trends in Amplification, Vol.2, No.2, 1997, Development of Digital Hearing Aids by Christopher Schweitzer, Ph.D. Woodland Publications, Inc., New York, NY (212)566-4294

Fig. 19-3 Progression of a Binary Code as contrast to the more familiar Decimal System

THE AMPLIFICATION PROCESS OF THE DSP HEARING INSTRUMENT

Figure 19-4 shows a basic block diagram of a DSP hearing instrument. The following sections will reference the blocks in the diagram to illustrate how a digital hearing instrument processes the signal.

MICROPHONE AND PRE-AMP (INPUT STAGE)

The microphone used in a DSP hearing instrument is the same as that used in an analog hearing instrument. It's function is to convert the incoming sound to an electrical signal. Following the microphone there is usually some form of amplification applied to the signal. This is done with the Pre-amp (Pre-amplifier). Typically, this amplification is on the order of 10-15dB, but it can be higher.

ANALOG-TO-DIGITAL CONVERSION

The signal must now be converted from an analog signal to a digital format of binary numbers. This conversion is performed by the analog-to-digital converter, and it involves two processes: Sampling and Quantization.

The sampling rate, which determines frequency resolution, refers to how often the waveform amplitude is measured. The signal from the microphone is not processed as a continuous signal, but is sampled at discrete intervals. The sampling process involves the generation of a train of pulses that capture the amplitude at each of these intervals. The more frequently the sampling pulses occur, the more samples will be obtained within a given period of time. Thus, more detail of the changes occurring over time can be captured with a higher sampling rate. In a digital hearing instrument with a sampling rate of 16kHz, the instantaneous value of the sine wave is measured 16,000 times per second. The sampling rate has a direct bearing on the frequency bandwidth that can be accurately represented.

The Nyquist theorem is a basic rule of digital sampling which states that the sampling rate must be at least twice as fast as the highest frequency that is desired in the signal processing. This minimum frequency is called the Nyquist frequency. It is defined as one-half the sampling rate. If, for example, you want to represent frequencies up to 8kHz, the sampling rate would need to be at least 16kHz, and 8kHz would be the Nyquist frequency. If a frequency component higher than the Nyquist frequency is sampled, a type of error known as aliasing will occur. When aliasing occurs, the higher frequencies that are greater than one-half the sampling rate, may appear as different lower frequencies when sampled. This "folding-over" of high frequencies into lower frequencies introduces erroneous components into the signal. If not properly handled, these signals may be audible as distortion in the final output signal. To avoid aliasing errors, an analog low-pass filter, called an anti-aliasing filter, is placed prior to the A/D converter to prohibit introduction of frequency components that are higher than the Nyquist frequency. Figure 19-5 provides a simple illustration of aliasing.

The second process, Quantization, refers to how finely the amplitude variations are measured, and is reported as the number of bits used in the conversion process. The amplitudes of the waveform at the sampled points are converted into digits. For each sampled point, a digital value is assigned that corresponds to the appropriate region. Figure 19-6 provides an illustration of the sampling and analog-to-digital conversion process.

The number of bits, sometimes referred to as "wordwidth", defines the amplitude resolution or amplitude detail of the signal. As a general rule, the faster the sampling rate and the greater the number of bits, the closer the digital signal will be to the original analog signal, when it is converted back into an analog signal. The number of bits also impact the dynamic range of the hearing instrument. The dynamic range is the difference between the ongoing noise floor of the instrument and the onset of saturation at the upper end. Each bit contributes approximately 6dB to the dynamic range, so increasing the number of bits, improves the dynamic range of the instrument. For example, a 16 bit system would have a dynamic range of 96dB (16x6). As a comparison, most linear analog hearing instruments have an effective dynamic of about 60dB.

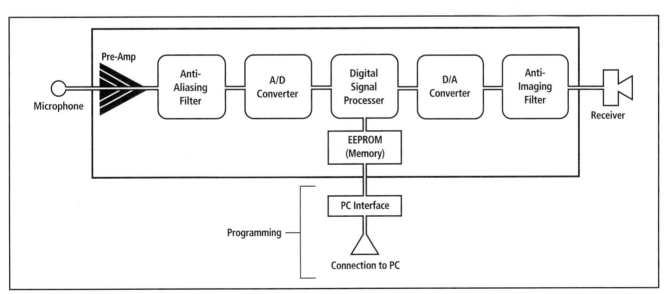

Fig. 19-4 Basic Block of a DSP Hearing Instrument

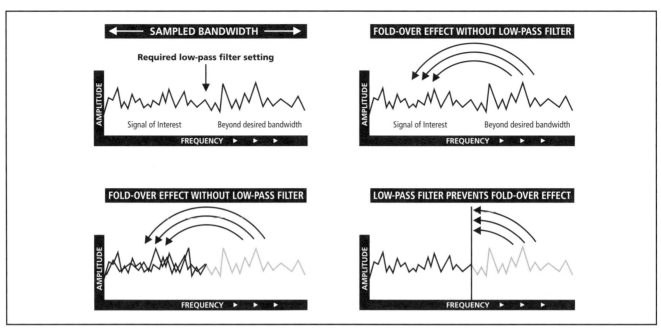

Fig. 19-5 Illustration of Aliasing

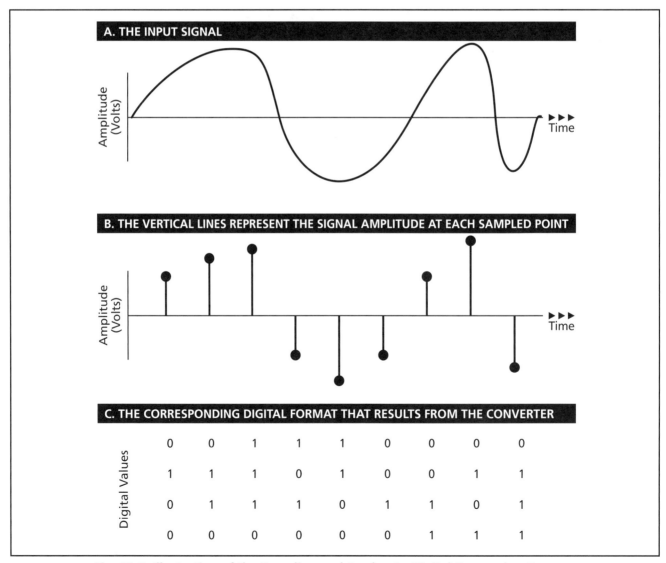

Fig. 19-6 Illustration of the Sampling and Analog to Digital Conversion Process

19-6

At the time of this writing, parameters for analog-to-digital conversion in hearing instruments consist of sampling rates of at least 16kHz and bit rates of at least 16 bits. The encoding of the digital signal with these parameters should be sufficient enough for good frequency and amplitude resolution.

The type of A/D converter that is presently considered the best technique for use in digital audio products, including hearing instruments, is the Sigma-Delta converter. The Sigma-Delta converter makes use of a very high sampling rate, often referred to as oversampling. The signal is actually sampled hundreds of thousands or even millions of times per second and converted to a robust one bit stream. Then, the signal is re-converted to a more conventional digital signal, such as a 16kHz, 16 bit signal, for digital processing operations.

Figure 19-7 illustrates the approach used with one popular DSP hearing instrument in which the signal is first converted to a 1MHz, 1 bit stream, then re-converted to a final 32kHz, 20 bit signal.

It is important to note that regardless of the sampling and bit rates utilized, the performance and frequency limits that are achievable with digital hearing instruments will be limited by the transducers, i.e. microphones and receivers. For example, the frequency response of the receiver will restrict the hearing instrument performance more than the analog-to-digital conversion process. Even though the frequency limit of the digital circuit is defined by the sampling rate, increasing the sampling rate will not extend the entire system response beyond what the receiver is capable of achieving.

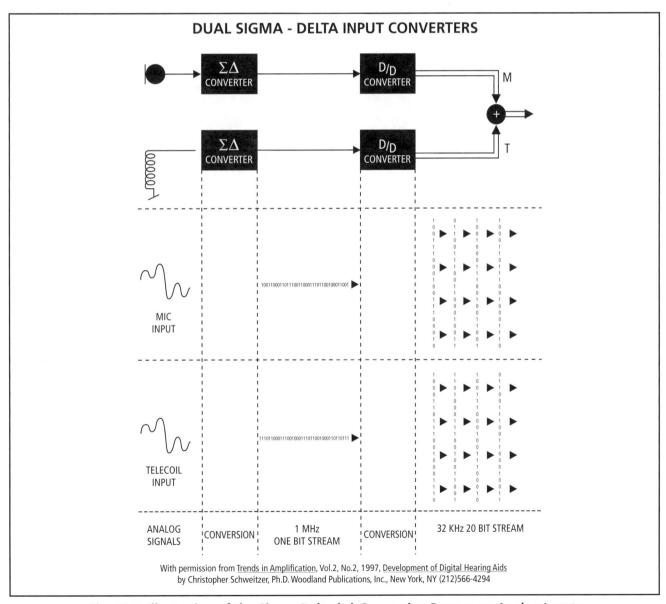

DUAL SIGMA - DELTA INPUT CONVERTERS

With permission from Trends in Amplification, Vol.2, No.2, 1997, Development of Digital Hearing Aids
by Christopher Schweitzer, Ph.D. Woodland Publications, Inc., New York, NY (212)566-4294

**Fig. 19-7 Illustration of the Sigma-Delta ( ) Conversion Process on Analog Inputs
from either the Microphone or Telecoil in a DSP Hearing Instrument**

DIGITAL SIGNAL PROCESSOR

Next in the process is the digital signal processor. The digital signal processor is the heart of the DSP hearing instrument. the sole reason for the analog-to-digital conversion process is to transform the signal into a useable form for the processor. It is the "computer" within the hearing instrument that, according to the specified algorithm, performs mathematical operations on the digitized signal that define the signal processing. An algorithm is a list of rules or instructions for processing the signal. Filtering, multiple-band compression, noise reduction, and speech enhancement are types of algorithms that might be accomplished by the microprocessor. The digital signal processor must be capable of processing thousands and thousands of instructions at high speeds. All of the processing, including the A/D conversion, must be performed in a fraction of a second. The processing algorithm is what will typically differentiate one digital hearing instrument from another.

The memory (EEPROM) stores the processing parameters and allows a programming instrument to change them. Several different types of programmers are in use. The most common is the use of a combination fitting and programming system that runs on a personal computer.

For programming, the hearing instrument and the PC communicate via an interface box which plugs into the computer. At the time of this writing, an interface box called HiPro, is most commonly used. The hearing instrument connects to the PC interface through a cable with a special "battery pill" that is inserted into the battery compartment of the hearing instrument, or with a subminiature plug that is inserted into a corresponding socket on the hearing instrument.

DIGITAL-TO-ANALOG CONVERSION AND OUTPUT STAGE

Following the DSP operations, the digital signal must be converted back into an analog signal. The digital-to-analog converter essentially reverses the operation performed by the analog-to-digital converter to change the signal back from numbers into a waveform. At this stage, changes occur abruptly, artificially introducing high frequency energy into the signal. These erroneous high frequency components, called "images", occur at values above the Nyquist frequency, and can be audible if they are not properly handled. A low-pass filter, referred to as an anti-imaging filter, is used to prevent this problem. The signal is then passed to the receiver, where the conversion to an audible analog signal is completed.

An alternative approach that is used for digital-to-analog conversion eliminates the need for a discrete D/A converter. This approach has been called Direct Digital Drive. The digital signal is passed directly from the DSP processor to a digital output driver and to the receiver, for both the low-pass filtering and demodulation into an audible analog signal. This approach saves both power consumption and physical space in the hearing instrument.

OPEN-FIT AND SEALED-FIT MINI BTE HEARING AIDS

L E S S O N   20

BACKGROUND/DESCRIPTIONS

Behind-the-Ear open-fit (with speaker in-aid – SIA) and speaker-in-ear canal (SIE) hearing aid styles are a recent, rapid growth phenomenon, but are not new to hearing aid dispensing. Open fittings evolved from small vents originally intended to reduce pressure sensation concerns, then larger to about 2 mm+ diameter to produce usable low-frequency suppression to assist high-frequency losses and reduction of occlusion and the occlusion effect, to tubing only. Speaker-in-the-ear canal included body-worn and early BTE hearing aids.

Collectively, these recent iterations of early style hearing aids are referred to as Mini BTE hearing aids, with the styles identified as:

1.   SIA-O   Speaker-in-Aid (Open Fit)
2.   SIE-O   Speaker-in-Ear (Open Fit)
3.   SIE-S   Speaker-in-Ear (Sealed Fit)

SIA-O (SPEAKER-IN-AID–OPEN)

In this style, sound emanates from a speaker in the hearing aid and is directed into the ear canal via a fine hollow plastic tube. Inside the ear canal a small, soft silicone dome or molded, vented acrylic tip holds the tube in place (Fig. 20-1).

SIE-O (SPEAKER-IN-EAR–OPEN)

This style open-fit hearing aid utilizes an external speaker that is placed inside the ear canal (RIE – Receiver-In-Ear; or SIE – Speaker-In-Ear), being connected to the processor by a thin wire. The speaker is encased in a silicone dome or molded acrylic tip with venting of sufficient size to allow the ear canal to remain essentially "open," or what is identified as SIE-O (Fig. 20-2).

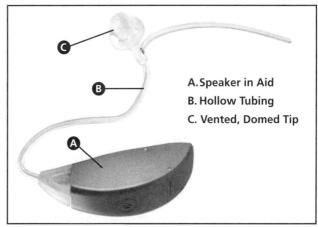

A. Speaker in Aid
B. Hollow Tubing
C. Vented, Domed Tip

Fig. 20-1 Speaker-in-aid (open fit) hearing aid. Used by permission of GN ReSound.

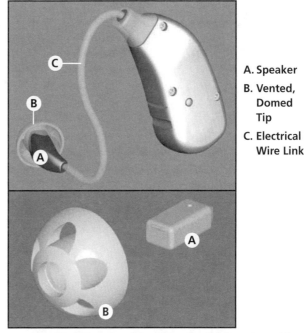

A. Speaker
B. Vented, Domed Tip
C. Electrical Wire Link

Fig. 20-2 Speaker-in-ear (open fit) hearing aid. Used by permission of Siemans Hearing Instruments.

SIE-S
(SPEAKER-IN-EAR – SEALED)

In this iteration the speaker is encased in a tip that provides a "seal" (closed fit) to provide for (a) maximum acoustical benefits and (b) efficiencies in order to fit more severe hearing losses (Fig. 20-3).

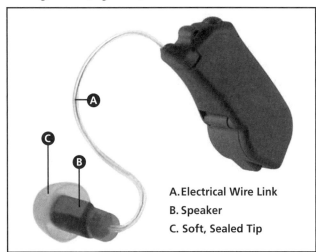

A. Electrical Wire Link
B. Speaker
C. Soft, Sealed Tip

Fig. 20-3 Speaker-in-ear (sealed fit) hearing aid. Used by permission of SeboTek Hearing Systems.

A major difference between the SIA and SIE designs is that in the latter, the sound processor is allowed to be of even smaller size because the speaker is no longer encased in it, but in the ear canal. The tips used with these fittings are flexible and available in various sizes to ensure optimal comfort.

GENERAL FITTING ADVANTAGES

The advantages of SIA and SIE fittings are that they provide:

- Cosmetic improvement (smaller size and thin tubing, or wire, render the instrument essentially "invisible" when worn)

- Comfort of fit due to conformability of ear pieces of various sizes, shapes, and materials

- Enhanced opportunity to fit less severe hearing losses satisfactorily (first-time users and younger-age users due to cosmetic acceptance)

- Same-session fittings and service

- Removal of the custom earmold, which has consistently been identified as a major fitting problem area

- Improved efficiency in the dispensing office (less time involved because of the elimination of ear impressions, earmolds, earmold remakes, and shell modifications)

- An immediate opportunity for the patient to experience the final fit (cosmetics, sound, comfort)

- Action on electroacoustics rather than the mechanics of the earmold

- Simplified fitting and use, but adjustable to meet patient needs

- Modular concept for inventory control and repair

SPECIFIC FITTING ISSUES – SIA FIT

SIA hearing aids are designed primarily to reduce the sensation that the ear(s) are plugged (occluded) when hearing aids are worn, and also to reduce the occlusion effect (the sensation of one's voice being too loud when speaking, chewing, etc.) when hearing aid earmolds are improperly fitted.

The large venting created by such fittings bypasses low-frequency amplification, leaving more of what is being amplified in the higher frequencies. As a result, these open-fit hearing aids are most often recommended for individuals having relatively normal or near-normal hearing in the low frequencies and a mild-to-moderate sloping high-frequency loss. The caveat is that the open canal increases the likelihood of feedback, and as such, limits the severity of hearing loss that can be fitted. Without a feedback reduction/cancellation circuit, the maximum gain is approximately 20 dB. Note that without feedback management, of the patients seen with the average audiometric configuration in Fig. 20-4, 1/3 could not have been fitted with an open mold.

Fortunately, technology has allowed open fittings (SIA and SIE-O instruments) to control this major fitting limitation. Essentially all are fitted to patients with some type of feedback cancellation system designed to minimize or eliminate acoustic feedback, allowing approximately 10 dB additional gain prior to the onset of feedback. These open-fit instruments keep the ears open to sound, rather than plugging the ear with the physical hearing aid or earmold. The lower-pitched sounds that do not require amplification, such that the sound of one's own voice travel normally through the ear canal, remaining natural and comfortable.

Although there are countless numbers of successful fittings, there still remain those that are not successful. Several issues related to open fittings specifically may be responsible for most of these failures. For example, one of the primary reasons for a resurgence of open fittings is the availability of feedback cancellation (FBC) techniques (allowing more gain). However, these do not guarantee a feedback-free fitting. How much more gain is achievable varies widely and depends on the capabilities of the FBC algorithm.

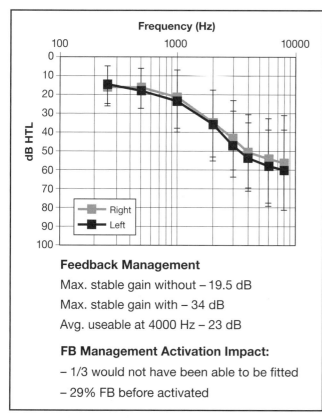

Feedback Management

Max. stable gain without – 19.5 dB

Max. stable gain with – 34 dB

Avg. useable at 4000 Hz – 23 dB

FB Management Activation Impact:

– 1/3 would not have been able to be fitted

– 29% FB before activated

Fig. 20-4 SIA open-fit hearing aid applicable gains for the illustrated hearing loss shows that the maximum stable gain before feedback to be 19.5 dB, with a feedback cancellation algorithm, about 35 dB.

A second potential issue may be related to the amount of gain prescribed. Prescriptive formulas were developed for the traditional hearing aid fitting (i.e. closed mold or with no more than a 3-4 mm vent). Although targets for open-fit hearing aids should work in theory, many patients complain about over-amplification.

SPECIFIC FITTING ISSUES – SIE FIT

When the hearing loss is more severe, when greater gain without feedback is required, when directional microphones are needed for SNR (signal-to-noise) enhancement, when more specific control of acoustics is desired, when a smooth frequency response is needed, or when telecoils are suggested, a practical solution has been the SIE. SIE instruments are based on placing the speaker where it can perform best – in the ear canal.

SIE-O has many of the same limitations as does the SIA because it is essentially an open fit, with the exception that the speaker is placed in the ear canal and the transducers (microphone and speaker) are separated to allow for slightly greater losses to be fit before feedback occurs.

SIE-S instruments utilize an acoustic seal that performs two functions. (1) The seal, especially if more deeply in the ear canal, provides an acoustic overall increase in sound pressure level (SPL), especially in the high frequencies leading to increased hearing aid headroom. This added "gain" of approximately 20 dB allows the user to function with a reduced sound pressure from the hearing aid, and also (2) limits acoustic feedback, naturally. The seal of the fit also provides protection against loud sounds, something that an open fit cannot do because it allows these to enter unimpeded. And, if the seal is performed in the bony portion of the ear canal, the occlusion effect is reduced/eliminated, even though the ear canal is sealed. This style hearing aid allows for an extremely wide hearing loss fitting range - from wide band with extended high-frequency range for improved fidelity, low-frequency, high-frequency, and more severe hearing losses. And, the better the seal, the less feedback, with greater amplification available. A sealed earpiece eliminates phase interactions found in open fittings and requires no vent compensation strategy. It also results in less masking by ambient noises/sounds from entering the ear canal. Noise canceling algorithms are more likely to function properly, as will directionality (when implemented), and the frequency response of the aid is more properly determined because phase issues are not involved. The soft seal tip eliminates problems associated with custom-molded earpieces.

ISSUES SURROUNDING SIA AND SIE FITTINGS

1. **Feedback in hearing aids is managed using four primary approaches:**

   1. Static notch filters (signal audibility is compromised)

   2. Adaptive notch filters (a continuous monitoring of the feedback frequency with adjusting notch filters accordingly)

   3. Feedback suppression (estimates the feedback path as a function of frequency, then creates a digital filter with the same response. This digital filter is then applied to the signal-processing path in parallel. Where the feedback and the digital filter meet, there is subtraction, or no feedback signal. This can occur rapidly or slowly)

   4. Separate the transducers (this is the best solution for basic feedback reduction without any signal compromise). This approach is used with SIE approaches, and functions best with SIE-S, rather than SIE-O fittings.

2. The Vent as a two-channel device

A vent in an earpiece allows for two channels of activity. The first is a feedback channel where the sound escaping through the vent is reamplified by the microphone, regardless of where the microphone is placed (in the ear or over the ear). The second channel allows sound not transmitted through the tympanic membrane to escape outwardly through the vent, resulting in a phase delay with the incoming signal being directed inwardly through the vent (Fig. 20-5).

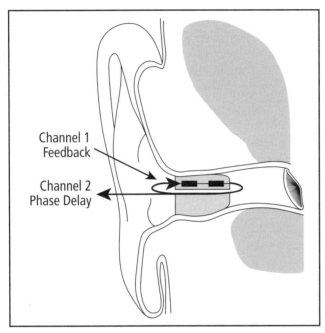

Fig. 20-5 The hearing aid vented earpiece illustrating that it functions as a two-channel device, which is not desirable.

3. Phase (time)

Phase has an impact on the performance of a hearing aid. It can cause unwanted resonances and cancellations of the incoming signal, depending on how the aid is coupled to the ear. Some resonances will cause "ringing," feedback, or generate distortions. As such, phase can have a negative impact on open fittings, directional microphone fittings, noise cancellation algorithms, and on the "expected" programming algorithm results associated with an open fitting.

With an open fitting, sounds at the eardrum arrive directly through the open vent and from the hearing instrument as an amplified signal. These two different sounds interact with each other (phase differences), and may compromise sound quality, audibility, and word recognition (Fig. 20-6). In some cases attempts are made to 'coordinate' these two different sounds. With a sealed fitting, the only signal is that from the hearing aid and phase effects from a vent are not an issue.

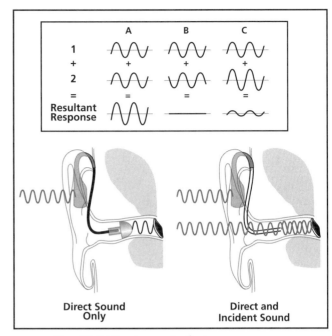

Fig. 20-6 The impact of phase on open-versus sealed-fit hearing aids.

In the case of the open-fit, the sound arrives at the eardrum at two different times, with some of the reflected sound from the eardrum interacting with the open ear incoming sound in unpredictable ways. In the sealed-fit condition, only one sound is directed to the eardrum.

4. Processing Time (Relative to Time and Phase Management)

Digital Signal Processing (DSP) hearing aids experience a delay during the analog to digital exchange. Delay, especially if longer than 5 msec, has a direct effect on sound quality, and if longer than 15 msec. can be experienced as an echo. When present, such "echoes" are often confused with "hollowness of sound" and contribute to sound quality complaints. When associated with an open-fit, delays introduce additional phase interactions.

5. Tubing Effects

The tubing used to direct sound from the sound processor to the ear canal causes significant changes to the expected frequency response. The more tubing that exists, the greater are the peaks and valleys in the frequency response (plumbing effects resulting in an unsmoothed frequency response). A SIE instrument has a much smoother frequency response than a SIA because the SIE has essentially no tubing. Additionally, the inside diameter of the tubing on a SIA distorts the frequency response of the aid, especially in the high frequencies – the smaller the tubing diameter, the more the high frequencies are reduced (Fig. 20-7). And, the thinner the tubing wall thickness, the greater is the opportunity for acoustic feedback by sound leakage through the tube walls.

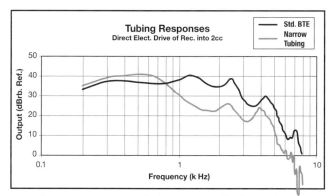

Fig. 20-7 In open-fit hearing aids the tubing diameter has a profound effect on the frequency response of the hearing aid.

5. Sealed (Closed) and Open-fit Insertion Gain Comparisons

With a sealed earpiece, greater sound pressure can be expected over an open fit. And, even more is expected with the speaker inserted more deeply.

The level of hearing aid gain required to overcome the insertion loss (IL) – often expressed as Real Ear Occluded Response (REOR) - created by a hearing aid earmold is clouded with many distortions.

In reality, the discussion of overcoming REOR (or an insertion loss) by a hearing aid's amplification is significant ONLY with vented fittings (including the extreme case of open fittings). The lower the REOR (greater insertion loss, as with a closed mold) the more the sound pressure in the ear canal is determined by the hearing aid alone, and is more predictable. With a closed mold the sound pressure in the ear canal can be predicted directly since there are no phase shifts due to differences between the incident sound and the amplified sound. In vented/open fittings, this prediction is confounded by unpredictable phase differences due to time of arrival of the incident and amplified sound. What happens in vented/open fittings is a bass drop-off as the coupling becomes more open and interaction occurs between the two sound pathways because the gains between them are approximately equal.

Additionally, evidence suggests that the practical, maximum stable high-frequency gain of an open-fit device is 30 dB.

6. Directional Microphone Performance

The benefits of directional microphone hearing aids are well understood and are maximum with SIE-S fittings. However, it has been shown that there is some benefit in the SNR (signal-to-noise ratio) with open-fit hearing aids, but not to the same degree as with a closed mold system.

7. Bandwidth and Its Relationship to Intelligibility and Gain

The wider the amplification bandwidth, the greater the intelligibility and the less sound pressure that is required to overcome a hearing loss. As the frequency response narrows (less lows and more high-frequency response, as seen in open-fit instruments), the greater the sound pressure has to be to achieve the same intelligibility. This is normally experienced as a demand for increased gain in the hearing aid on the part of the patient. SIE-S instruments are more likely to provide extended frequency response range, including extended high-frequency response.

PERFORMANCE VERIFICATION

The response shown on the hearing aid programming software and the 2-cc coupler responses on the hearing aid specification sheet are not accurate representations of how the hearing aid performs once coupled to the ear. For this, real-ear measurements are required. Figure 20-8 shows a comparison of 2-cc measurements versus real ear measurements of an open-fit hearing aid.

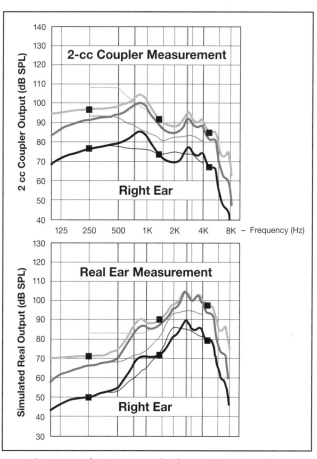

Fig. 20-8 The top graph shows 2-cc coupler responses in SPL and the lower graph shows the same open-fit hearing aid real-ear responses.

COUPLER MEASUREMENTS

Open-fit hearing aids do not easily adapt to the standard HA-1 and HA-2 couplers used for performing sound chamber measurements on hearing aids that fit snugly into the canal or that have attached earmolds. Attempts to use these couplers produce resulting frequency response curves nothing like the real-ear response of the hearing aid.

A special open-fit coupler has been designed that provides a realistic frequency response and makes it easy to attach the open-fit hearing aid to the coupler (Fig. 20-9). The open-fit tip is placed into the coupler as it would be placed into the patient's ear. This is not a standard 2-cc coupler and therefore cannot be used to compare to manufacturing specifications, but it will provide a much more realistic frequency response.

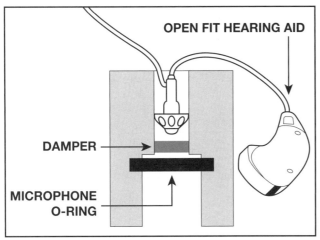

Fig. 20-9 Diagram of an open-fit measurement coupler.

REAL-EAR MEASUREMENTS

Real-ear verification for hearing aids is a necessary element of a hearing aid dispensing practice.

Real-ear measurements of SIE-S hearing aids can be performed normally. Open-fit hearing aids, however, can yield error results if not accounted for. While the error is not great, serious professionals should consider making a measurement adjustment if results are to be used for comparison purposes. The adjustment to be made is to deactivate the reference microphone when making the REAR (Real Ear Aided Response) measurement. Figure 20-10 shows the REAR measurement artifact at 2500 Hz with the reference microphone left on (curve 2) versus the reference microphone off (curve 3). Curve 1 is the REUR (Real Ear Unaided Response).

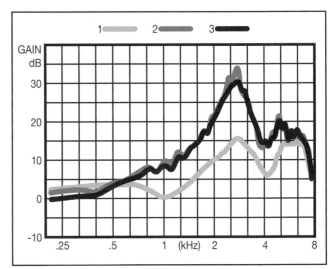

Fig. 20-10 Differences in open-fit real-ear results when the reference mic is not turned off when making REAR measurement.

HEARING INSTRUMENT HISTORY

LESSON 21

A hearing instrument is an ultra miniature electro-acoustical device that is always too large. It must amplify sounds a million times, but bring in no noise. It must operate, without failure, in a sea of perspiration, a cloud of talcum powder, or both. It is a product that one puts off buying for ten years after he needs it, but cannot do without it for thirty minutes when it has to be serviced.

Sam Lybarger

By cupping the hand behind the ear, sound is amplified by approximately 5 - 8 dB. By the early 1800's and 1900's, ear trumpets and horns of all shapes and sizes abounded. Some provided up to 15 dB of gain. All of these methods collected sound and funnelled it into the ear.

AMPLIFIED SOUND

Alexander Graham Bell invented the telephone in 1876. The **first patent** in 1892, was for a **telephone-type electric hearing instrument.** Manufactured in 1903, it remained commercially available 'til the 1930's. The instrument used a carbon granule microphone, a battery, and magnetic earphone. Its frequency range of 1000 Hz - 1800 Hz produced 10 - 15 dB gain.

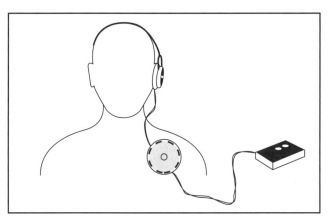

Fig. 20-1
Electric Hearing Instrument

A carbon microphone consists of two thin, carbon coated metal plates. One plate is pliable, forming a diaphragm. Sandwiched between the plates, and under slight pressure, are carbon balls, shots, granules or dust. With any body movement, like bending forward or leaning back, the granules shift, causing heavy static before the sound fades or shuts off entirely.

Larger hearing instruments with **vacuum tube** amplifiers heralded the 1920's. They had more gain and clarity, but were less wearable. Some were desk-size, others portable in small suitcases. The vacuum tube amplifies a signal by controlling voltage changes in a circuit.

Vacuum tubes require at least two batteries with different voltages. The filament generates heat. Europeans call the vacuum tube a **valve,** since it works like a valve in controlling electromotive force in a circuit.

Price-wise, todays' hearing instruments are the best deal in town. For instance, in 1923, the Western Electric Company produced their Model 10-A, with a complete binaural circuit. This gem, housed in a 1' x 3' x 4' cabinet, only weighed 222 lbs. Its price - $2,250.00, not including the automobile storage battery or installation.

Technological improvements reduced the weight to 135 lbs by 1929.

Vacuum tube amplifiers were compatable with a crystal **microphone** as both had a high impedance.

Wearable Hearing instruments: In 1938, a big turning point in hearing instrument development was the introduction of the **miniature vacuum tube.** This, along with the design and production of **small crystal receivers,** made a 'wearable' body worn electronic instrument possible.

Crystal microphones and receivers failed under high temperatures, couldn't withstand high humidity, and were very fragile. Magnetic microphones and receivers replaced crystal in vacuum tube hearing instruments.

Head Worn instruments: The **transistor**'s arrival in the early 1950's replaced the vacuum tube, making hearing instruments considerably smaller, more rugged, and longer lasting. The transistor amplifies by controlling current changes using only one low voltage battery.

Transistor amplifiers are compatable with **magnetic microphones** because both have low impedance. The magnetic microphone has a reasonably ideal frequency response over the speech range, but sacrificed very high and very low frequencies when it was miniaturized.

The **ceramic microphone,** a piezo-electrical microphone, improved on the crystal microphone. The high impedance of the ceramic microphone was a problem until the development of a FET (Field Effect Transistor), an impedance transforming device that also provides additional microphone sensitivity. It has extended low frequency amplification to 10 Hz, and is free of temperature and humidity problems. Damage from dropping is less than for the magnetic microphone.

The **integrated circuit (IC or 'chip'),** in 1964, consisted of transistors, resistors, and wiring on a tiny wafer of silicon. Now, with greater miniaturization, lower battery drain, and greater stability, future possibilities are endless.

The **electret microphone** replaced other microphones in most hearing instruments by 1982, and is presently in use. It is discussed further in 'Hearing Instrument Components and Characteristics', Lesson 22.

As the size of the transistor shrunk, so did other components - batteries, volume controls, microphones, receivers.

The Law of Conservation of Energy: Energy cannot be created or destroyed. Energy can be changed, converted or transduced from one form to another.

Two basic principles of electronics are critical to hearing instrument design - transduction and amplification.

TRANSDUCTION

Transducers change energy from one form to another. Acoustic energy is hard to control. If we transduce acoustic energy into an electrical signal, it is easier to change and modify.

A **microphone and receiver** transduce energy. The microphone changes acoustic energy, or sound waves, into electrical energy. We amplify and modify the electrical energy. Then, the receiver converts (transduces) it back to acoustic energy. The acoustic energy is modified again by the acoustic coupling of the earmold before the ear hears the sounds.

ELECTRICAL ENERGY

The flow of electricity requires a **positive and negative charge.**

Electrical energy uses the **atom,** the smallest part of any material. **Atoms are electrically neutral.** An atom has a central nucleus of **protons and neutrons,** with **electrons** orbiting around it. The electrons are arranged in shells, with two electrons in the inner shell. The outer shell **has room for eight electrons.**

Protons carry a positive charge.

Neutrons are electrically neutral, with no positive or negative charge.

Electrons carry a negative charge.

If an atom is electrically neutral, then the number of protons and electrons must be equal.

Basic Law

1. Like charges repel. Protons repel protons. Electrons repel electrons.

2. Opposite charges attract. A proton attracts an electron.

Amplification: Only electrons move from atom to atom. The flow of electrons is **current, measured in amperes.** Electrical energy flows more easily through some materials than others.

Conductors: **Electrons** move through a conductor. Conductors, like copper, gold, silver, and aluminum, have one or two electrons in the outer shell that are not tightly bound to the nucleus. These electrons can move freely.

Semi-Conductors: Semi-conductors only allow an easy flow of electrons under certain conditions. Semi-conductors have four electrons in their outer shell. A semi-conductor acts like a conductor when energy in the form of heat, light or an electric field is applied, causing electrons in the outer shell to move.

The amount of electrical charge in each proton and electron determines how much current will flow. Materials with a greater charge have a larger flow of electrons. Charged objects close together have a greater flow than when they are farther apart.

A greater flow of current in a hearing instrument produces more volume or intensity.

Battery: Battery strength is measured in **volts.** The **hearing instrument battery** provides the power source to increase the flow of current. This power source acts like a pump, separating and holding positive and negative charges into two separate terminals. As opposite charges attract, and only electrons move, the attraction draws electrons to the positive terminal, creating current flow.

Direct Current (DC): **Direct current** always flows in one direction to the positive terminal. A battery generates direct current.

Alternating Current (AC): **Alternating Current** flows in both directions. Electrons flow to the positive terminal until it is no longer positive. The negative terminal, losing the electrons that make it negative, becomes positive, causing the electrons to return. Alternating current has a cycle, just like sound waves. When this reversal occurs sixty times in one second, it generates a sixty cycle or sixty Hertz current. Alternating current and sound both have frequency, wavelength, and amplitude. Generators produce alternating current. A microphone is a common generator.

Resistance or Impedance: Electrical resistance (impedance), measured in **ohms,** restricts electron movement, causing electrical 'friction' between the moving electrons and the stationery atom. Friction produces heat. For instance, a toaster works on resistance.

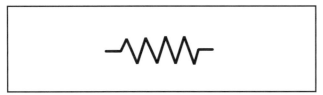

Fig. 21-1
Symbol for Resistors or Resistance

A resistor offers resistance **independant of frequency.**

The three major concepts using electricity are current, voltage, and resistance.

Ohm's Law

$$\text{Current} = \frac{\text{Voltage}}{\text{Resistance}}$$

OR

$$\text{Sound Pressure} = \frac{\text{Voltage (battery)}}{\text{Resistance}}$$

Current

1. Electrical current or sound pressure is directly proportional to the size of the voltage. Therefore, larger voltages produce greater currents or sound pressure levels.

2. Electrical current is inversely proportional to the resistance of a wire or tubing. Using larger wire or tubing results in less current.

Resistance

1. Resistance is directly proportional to length. A longer tubing or wire has more resistance **and emphasizes low frequencies. Shorter tubing or wire produces high frequency emphasis** because there is less resistance.

2. Resistance is inversely proportional to its cross-sectional area (width). Thicker wires or larger tubes offer less resistance because there is more room for the electrons or sound pressure to move. Wider tubing is less resistant, **allowing more high frequencies to flow freely.**

3. Materials have different resistances. Good **conductors** of electricity allow electrical energy to flow easily. **Semi-conductors,** like silicon or germanium, allow electricity to flow under certain conditions, but also have resistance characteristics.

Other materials, like plastics, glass, and rubber, cannot conduct electricity. Because they have such good **resistance,** they make excellent **insulators.** The outer shell of insulators is filled with electrons that are tightly bound to the nucleus.

Capacitors and Inductors: Capacitors and inductors, impede the flow of alternating current. They are measured in ohms, like resistors, but behave differently. Impedance describes them better than resistance.

A capacitor is essentially two metal plates, separated by a small distance.

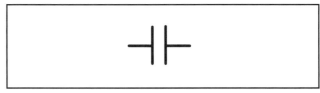

Fig. 21-2
Symbol for a Capacitor

The impedance of a capacitor decreases as the frequency of the alternating current decreases. A capacitor **passes the high frequencies and blocks the low frequencies.**

An inductor is made from a coiled wire. The impedance of an inductor increases as the alternating current increases. The flow of high frequency alternating current reduces with an inductor, **blocking the high frequencies and passing the lows.**

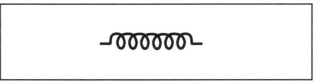

Fig. 21-3
Symbol for an Inductor

The combination of a capacitor and an inductor has minimal effect on the middle frequencies, but blocks both the lows and the highs.

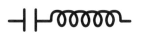

Fig. 21-4
Symbol for Capacitor and Inductor

Transistors: A transistor acts like a variable resistor, controlled by the input current. Small input current changes passing through the transistor produce large changes in the resistance of a circuit.

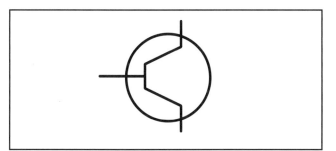

Fig. 21-5
Symbol for a Transistor

A transistor is a solid state semi-conductor, made of silicon. Adding an impurity to a semi-conductor is **'doping'.** The impurity lets a neighboring atom share the electrons in the outer shell, or 'attracts' electrons from the neighboring atoms.

Doping a semi-conductor with antimony, phosphorus, or arsenic creates an **n-type (negative)** semi-conductor, with an excess of electrons. Doping with boron, aluminum, or gallium creates a **p-type (positive)** semi-conductor with an electron deficiency.

An n-type semi-conductor sandwiched between two p-type semi-conductors produces positive-negative-positive (pnp) junctions. The middle of the sandwich is the **base,** and the outer portions are the **emitter** and **collector.** The deficiency of electrons created permits hole current.

Negative-positive-negative (npn) junctions sandwich the p-type semi-conductor in the middle. This creates an excess of electrons, permitting electron current.

Both electron current and hole current work in transistors for hearing instrument use.

Transistors are amplifiers. They allow current to pass in one direction only, and increase the flow of current passing through them. Transistors start almost instantly, are small, rugged, and have a long life.

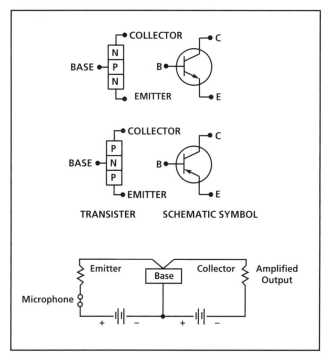

Fig. 21-6
Diagram of Transistor and
Simple Transistor Circuit

In hearing instruments, when the microphone transduces acoustic energy into electrical energy, this small input electrical energy passes through the transistor. The transistor converts the current from the battery into a large, desired output current. The input current to the transistor strongly influences the output current.

INTEGRATED CIRCUITS

An amplifier consisted of transistors, capacitors, resistors and switches. It was the largest, most complex part of the hearing instrument until the development of the integrated circuit (IC).

Each component in a hearing instrument either has its own frequency response characteristics or modifies the existing response in some way. The response curve of a hearing instrument is a combination of the response curves of each of the components. Technology is now at the point where it is possible to produce almost any electroacoustic response.

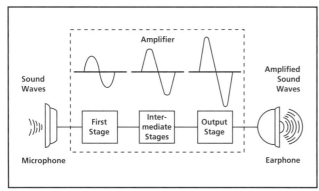

Fig. 22-1
Basic Hearing Aid Circuit

Transducers: A **microphone is an input transducer,** changing or transducing acoustic energy to mechanical energy, then to electrical energy. Electrical energy is easier to adjust or modify than acoustic energy, producing a signal that benefits the communication of the patient.

The **receiver, an output transducer,** converts or transduces the modified electrical signal back to acoustic energy. Earmold acoustics also modify the energy before the patient hears the sound.

Microphones: Microphones have a frequency response. The electret microphone is the most versatile microphone for hearing instrument use, replacing most other microphones by 1982. Virtually all fields of audio amplification, recording and communications use electret microphones. Their use is not limited to hearing instruments.

Magnetic, ceramic, and electret microphones are **omni-directional microphones,** receiving sound equally well in all directions. They are classified by physical design - magnetic, ceramic, or electret.

Electret Microphone: An **electret microphone** is not really a microphone, but a piece of permanently polarized material. It has a wide, flat frequency response, with excellent sensitivity and durability. The diaphragm is the only moving part. Electret condenser microphone is technically correct, but seldom used.

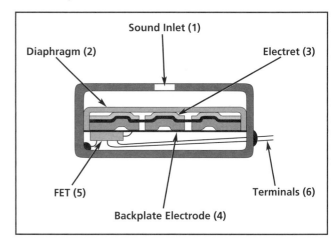

Fig. 22-2
Electret Condenser Microphone

In the cutaway diagram above, sound enters the microphone case (1). The sound waves in compression and rarefaction easily vibrate a thin diaphragm (2) made of a negatively charged foil sensing surface. The vibrating diaphragm transduces acoustic energy to mechanical energy. The diaphragm puts pressure on the electret (3), mounted on the conducting back plate electrode (4). Both the underside of the diaphragm and the backplate connect to a Field Effect Transistor (FET) preamplifier (5) with external terminals (6). As the diaphragm vibrates, the distance between the diaphragm and the backplate varies. The capacity of the diaphragm and backplate changes, resulting in voltage fluctuations which pass to the FET. The mechanical energy of the vibrating diaphragm transduces to an electrical signal. The signal travels to the external terminals, then to the amplifier.

Directional microphones, classified by their polar pattern, are more responsive to sound from the front than from behind.

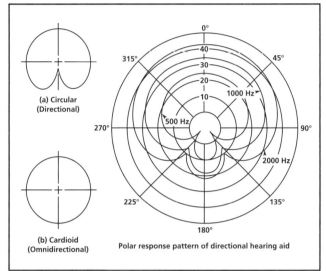

**Fig. 22-3
Polar Pattern Comparison of Directional and Omni-Directional Microphones**

A directional electret microphone has two openings or ports, one on each side of the diaphragm. The motion of the diaphragm depends on pressure differences from each port, using phase relationships.

Placement of the Microphone: Microphone placement, both in the hearing instrument, itself, and its relationship to the sound source, affect the perceived frequency response to the patient.

Receivers: The receiver is like a microphone in reverse. The electrical signal transduces to acoustic energy in the receiver.

As the electrical signal enters a magnetic field, the alternations in the signal cause a diaphragm to vibrate, setting up an acoustic signal.

Several receivers are presently in use. Most **air conduction receivers** are **internal,** built into the hearing instrument in behind-the-ear, in-the-ear, and canal models. Body-worn hearing instruments use **external receivers.** An external receiver attaches to a body-worn instrument by a cord, and clamps into a standard earmold.

Receivers have a resonant frequency, the frequency where they are most efficient.

Acoustic damping and earmold modifications have significant effects, smoothing out the sharp peaks in the frequency response of a hearing instrument. Acoustic damping is usually a filter, placed in the ear hook of the hearing instrument, or in the earmold tubing, itself. The closer the filter is to the ear canal, the greater the damping effect. Earmold modifications change the frequency response of the instrument too. This is covered more completely in the Earmolds lesson.

Bone conduction receivers are used with body-worn instruments, ear-level instruments, or the temple of hearing instrument glasses, where atresia or other conductive factors contraindicate the use of earmolds.

Amplifiers: Amplifiers increase the strength or intensity of electrical impulses from the microphone. Until the development of the Integrated Circuit (IC), the amplifier was the largest section of the hearing instrument with transistors, capacitors, resistors and switches.

Typically, amplifiers use three or more stages to provide accuracy, flexibility and stability. **Coupling** connects one stage in the amplifier to another. Although three or four stages are common, more is not better. The design of the circuit is important to the efficiency of transistors.

INTEGRATED CIRCUITS

The integrated circuit had the greatest impact on the electronics industry. An integrated circuit amplifier combines dozens of transistors and other components in layers on a tiny wafer of silicon. The components interconnect to perform various operations on electrical signals. Appropriate connections for parts that cannot be built in to the circuit are included - like capacitors (too large to incorporate), the microphone, battery, volume control and receiver.

Hybrid Circuits: Hybrid circuits incorporate even more components on the tiny silicon wafer, including several integrated circuits.

Fidelity is the ability to reproduce the signal as accurately as possible. Removing some of the original signal, or adding other frequencies, causes lack of fidelity in the amplified signal.

Amplifiers maintain the frequency response of the microphone. All amplifiers generate some form of distortion. Controlled frequency distortion is desirable, altering the frequency response to benefit the patient. Even our choice of microphone alters the frequency response from the way normal ears hear it. A good amplifier produces a large, completely accurate, undistorted copy of the input signal from the microphone.

Basic Linear Amplifiers: A linear amplifier amplifies the input sound at a constant rate until the amplifier reaches a natural limit and saturates or overloads, causing distortion.

The entire circuit, including the receiver, microphone, and battery voltage, determines the saturation output level. All electrical instruments have an inherent signal level, and cease linear operation above this level. Receivers reach overdrive limits faster than microphones.

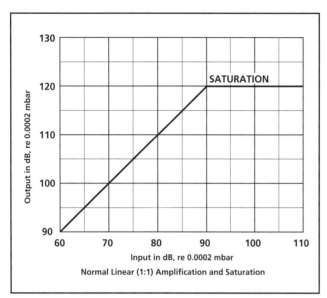

Fig. 22-4
Linear Input-Output Relationship

A linear amplifier has a 1:1 relationship. When the input sound increases 1 dB, then the output changes by 1 dB. The hearing instrument has a constant gain.

INPUT	+	GAIN	=	OUTPUT
60	+	30	=	90
70	+	30	=	100
80	+	30	=	110
90	+	30	=	120 * Saturation
100	+	30	=	120 *

A linear input, output curve (I/O) **always maintains a 45° slope** until the limit of the amplifier is reached. A line flatter than 45° is some form of compression. In the example above, the gain of the amplifier remains constant at 30 dB over the range of input signals from 60 dB to 90 dB. When the input increases to 100 dB, exceeding the saturation level of the amplifier, no output increase occurs.

SSPL 90, or MPO, measurements of the upper limit level in a hearing instrument, directly apply to **UCL** on the patient.

Although the amplifier has a natural limiting effect, artificial limiting is desirable. For example, this amplifier no longer gets louder above 120 dB SPL. If the patient has a

UCL of only 110 dB SPL, we want to limit the amplifier below natural saturation. The class of hearing instrument amplifier determines the method of limiting the output of the hearing instrument.

CLASSES OF AMPLIFIERS

Class A - Single Ended Amplifier

A Class A amplifier has a linear 1:1 I/O relationship. It uses only one output amplifier stage with one output transistor.

The method of limiting the amplifier output is **peak clipping.** Class A amplifiers use **non-symmetrical or hard peak clipping.** Resistors, connected in series with the receiver, vary the clipping or saturation level. Unsymmetrical peak clipping restricts half the sound wave.

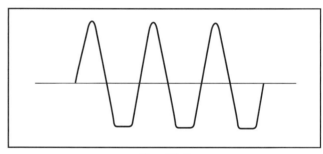

Fig. 22-5
Unsymmetrical Peak Clipping

Unsymmetrical peak clipping produces both odd and even harmonics, resulting in significant second order harmonic distortion, unpleasant sound reproduction, and loss of discrimination. Peak clipping limits the output instantaneously, but distortion results.

The advantage to peak clipping is circuit simplicity, where a few components accomplish instant output limiting in very little space. The hearing instrument maintains linear amplification over a wide range of input levels and still copes with output limiting directly.

The primary disadvantage is harmonic distortion, occurring above the limiting level.

A Class A amplifier works in mild to moderate output instruments, with an average output below 125 dB SPL.

Class B - Push-Pull Amplifier

Class B amplifiers are also linear, with a 1:1 input/output relationship and, again, the I/O graph is at a 45° angle. A line flatter than 45° is some form of compression.

The output stage uses a push-pull circuit for symmetrical peak clipping. Two transistors operate side by side, with two circuits rather than one. The first pushes and the second pulls the signal, producing only odd harmonics which have less affect on discrimination.

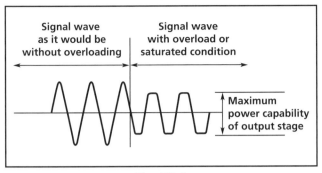

Fig. 22-6
Symmetrical Peak Clipping

Two transistors develop more current at the receiver, creating 6 dB more power (twice the intensity). Hearing instruments have an output greater than 125 dB SPL.

Artificial limiting of a Class B receiver also regulates a preselected output level, either by click adjustments or a potentiometer setting, and gain reduces at saturation.

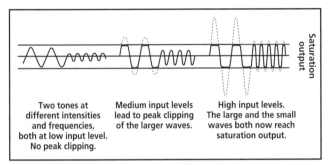

Fig. 22-7
Diagram Showing Various Degrees of Output 'Peak Clipping' with Different Levels of Input Signals

Push-pull circuits have the advantage of less distortion, more power, and higher gain. The disadvantage is battery current drain levels depend on the gain setting and background noise.

A linear instrument with peak clipping provides protection against sudden impact noises provided the MPO control is at least 12 dB louder than normal conversational levels.

SOFT PEAK CLIPPING or PEAK ROUNDING

When the method of limiting changes the output from a 1:1 relationship to less than a 45° angle, some form of **output compression** occurs. Soft peak clipping or peak rounding uses capacitors, diodes or variable resistors **at the output stage, after the volume control,** and between the last amplifier and receiver.

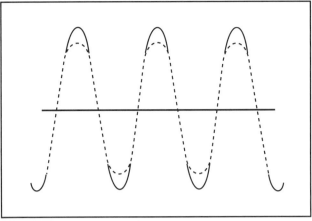

Fig. 22-8
Peak Rounding

Manufacturers' descriptions include diode clipping, diode compression control, modified peak clipping, peak rounding, soft peak clipping, output compression, etc. Each **limits the output of the hearing instrument** in a non-linear fashion.

Although part of the range of the instrument is linear, the I/O graph varies from a 45° angle at the fitter adjustable point. The non-linearity gradually reduces the output as the input increases. The **knee-point** is where the signal changes from linear to non-linear amplification.

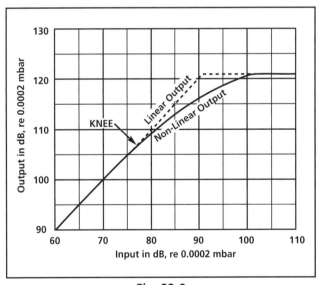

Fig. 22-9
Non-Linear Peak Rounding I/O Curve

Peak clipping is instantaneous. Non-linear output limiting, when the input sound reaches the specified intensity, is gradual as the intensity increases. Non-linearity causes harmonic distortion from the point where the I/O curve varies from the 45° angle, but the distortion is not as severe as unsymmetrical hard peak clipping.

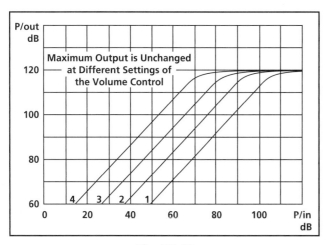

Fig. 22-10
Output Compression Input - Output Characteristics at 2000 Hz at Different Volume Control Settings

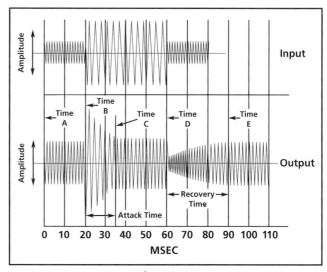

Fig. 22-11
Attack and Release Time

COMPRESSION AMPLIFIERS

Compression amplifiers are not instant. They have a **time delay feedback loop before the volume and tone controls,** measuring and controlling the **input** sound.

There are two methods of controlling compression, input and output. Both involve the use of feedback circuits to accomplish the method of control. With input compression the feedback loop monitors the instrument circuit just after the microphone. The feedback loop returns the signal to the amplifier 180 degrees out of phase to the input signal.

Output compression monitors the signal after the amplifier and before the signal reaches the receiver. The signal is returned to the amplifier 180 degrees out of phase with the primary signal.

Changes in the volume control with input compression will reduce the knee-point for the compression level. This provides two way protection for the patient. Input compression preserves the S/N (signal-to-noise) ratio. Changes in the volume control level with output compression will not reduce the knee-point for the compression level. The feedback circuit operates with 'attack' and 'release' time delays.

Attack Time: Attack time is the delay required for the feedback loop to recognize and act upon a loud input signal. Attack time ceases when the amplifier reaches a quieter steady state.

The top section graphically shows a signal at normal volume, then a loud sound. When the loud sound ceases, the signal returns to normal again.

The bottom section demonstrates how the feedback loop in an AGC circuit works. Time A to time B shows the normal amplified signal. The loud sound starts at time B, but it takes a few milliseconds before the amplifier compresses the loud sound to an acceptable level. The distance from time B to time C is attack time.

Loud sounds 'overshoot' during this time delay period, so ideally the attack time should be short - 2 to 10 milliseconds. A faster attack time reacts on individual phonemes in a single word, creating a flutter or pumping sound. Some hearing instruments use peak clipping to control the intensity of the overshoot.

Release Time: At time D, the loud sound ceases. Now the feedback loop must reverse the compression procedure and return the 'undershoot' to normal amplification. The milliseconds taken between time D and time E allow the amplifier to recover or release the compressed signal.

When the input sound becomes quieter, release time is the feedback delay before the amplifier no longer compresses the signal, and it returns to the normal steady state. If the release time is too slow, the signal appears to 'black out' or flutter because the quiet signal is too quiet in compression. A release time of 50 - 100 milliseconds is recommended.

When limiting is lowered from the natural SSPL of the hearing instrument, fluctuation becomes more noticeable and may overcome the advantages of lower limiting levels.

There are two types of compression amplifiers with a **fixed frequency response** - Automatic Gain Control (AGC) and Logarithmic Compression.

AGC - High Level Compression: When **a feedback circuit controls amplifier gain,** Automatic Gain Control (AGC) is the electrical term, and Automatic Volume Control (AVC) is the acoustical term. The volume control setting determines the output of the hearing instrument. The MPO control sets the peak clipping 'overshoot' at the output.

Although you can turn down the volume control to reduce gain on an output compression instrument, an AGC feedback network adjusts the output faster and more accurately than a manual volume control adjustment.

Sounds are not cut off, like peak clipping. The strongest signals entering the circuit trigger an additional circuit and part of the excess energy feeds back in opposition to the signal. This causes a gain reduction at high levels.

Amplitude is linear at all AGC settings in the same way as if we turn the volume control down manually. Whether the signal is high frequency or low frequency, the complex wave reduces across all frequencies.

Other terms are High Level Compression, Curvilinear AGC, Linear AGC, Automatic Level Control. The effort to control attack and release times produces a curvilinear I/O curve. The knee-point is set above normal conversational levels.

Logarithmic Compression - Low Level Compression: The total dynamic range reduces into smaller dynamic range without altering amplitude relationships of the signal components, regardless of the input level. Soft intensities amplify more than loud sounds. Gain increases at low levels.

The I/O curve has less than 1:1 compression ratio, with a compression range of 5 - 25 dB.

A compression ratio compares the change in dB input SPL to the corresponding changes in output SPL. i.e., 30 dB input above the knee results in a 10 dB output SPL. the ratio is 3:1 or .33.

Low level compression changes with the input level and the frequency measured.

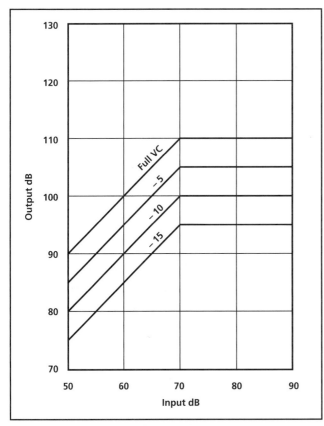

Fig. 22-12
Input - Output Characteristics at 2000 Hz
for anInput Compression Instrument

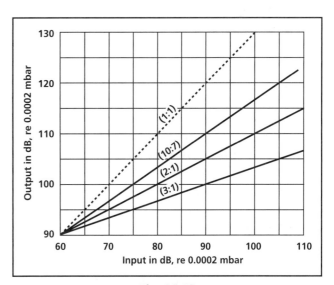

Fig. 22-13
Logarithmic Compression

Linear amplification changes to AGC (Automatic Gain Control) at the compression knee-point without significant Intermodulation or Harmonic Distortion. At any AGC activated setting, signals are not compressed in amplitude.

Since compression occurs at low input levels as well as near UCL, the knee-point is much lower than AGC compression. The knee is often the noticeable difference between AGC and logarithmic compression.

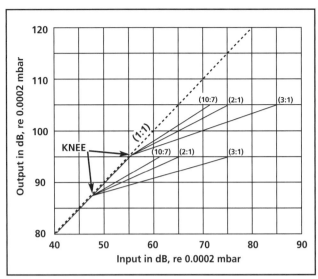

Fig. 22-14
I/O Comparision of AGC and
Logarithmic Compression

Logarithmic compression, Dynamic Range Compression, and Linear Dynamic Compression are examples of this type of compression.

AUTOMATIC SIGNAL PROCESSORS with LEVEL DEPENDENT FREQUENCY RESPONSE

Automatic signal processing (ASP) circuits perform tasks that patients find inconvenient, annoying, or impossible to do for themselves. The task of constantly adjusting the volume control led to the development of the AGC circuit. Adjusting a tone control leads to **level dependent frequency response (LDFR)** circuits, - multiple signal processors (MSP) and programmable hearing instruments - technology in its infancy.

Bill (Type 1): Low frequencies increase at quiet intensity levels and reduce at high intensity levels. The **environmental level of sound** determines the boost or cut in frequency response. This type of ASP describes the operation of circuits like the Manhattan circuit.

Till (Type 2): High frequencies increase at low levels and reduce at high levels. An example of this type of ASP is the K-AMP circuit. This circuit uses the new Class D amplifier and integrated receiver combination.

Pill (Type 3): Programmable instruments can reduce either lows, or highs, or both lows and highs - a combination of both Bill and Till, for example, ReSound and Ensoniq circuits.

Multiband signal processing instruments recognize differences in the input and frequency of incoming signals, and simultaneously adjust the competing audio spectrums of noise and speech. They divide the audio spectrum into more than one band. Each band has its own compression ratio. Each of its independent processing channels can ignore strong interference in another channel. The individual bands link together, but function independently.

Power Source (Battery): The battery is the power source that allows the amplifier to increase the input sound from the microphone. A weak battery limits the sound pressure possible in the hearing instrument.

The battery separates and holds the positive and negative charges onto two separate terminals. When an external wire connects the two terminals, electrical attraction draws the electrons to the positive terminal, creating current in the wire. The battery is usually a very small mercury or zinc-air cell. Although the cell is called a battery, the word battery means two or more cells used together.

Sometimes the power source is an 'accumulator', the correct term for a rechargeable cell, usually **nickel-cadmium (Nicad).** A nicad battery takes about fourteen hours to recharge.

Lithium batteries are used in programmable hearing instruments to hold the program constant.

Body-worn instruments use **alkaline batteries.**

Two batteries **connected in series,** i.e., positive to negative, give more power as the voltages are added. When both positives connect to one terminal, the cells **connect in parallel.** Voltages are not added. The total voltage is the same as the voltage of one cell. The useful life of the battery increases. Earlites and otoscopes use parallel connections.

Computing Battery Life: Battery current is measured in milliamperes, 1/1000 of an ampere.

Battery life = $\dfrac{\text{Battery capacity (mA hours)}}{\text{Battery current drain}}$

For example, if a battery is rated at 250 mA Hours, and the instrument requires a battery current of 2 mA, then the battery life is 125 hours.

$$\frac{250}{2} = 125 \quad OR \quad 250 \div 2 = 125$$

The electronics lesson discussed **components capable of changing or altering the gain or frequency response.**

Resistors offer resistance independant of frequency.

Capacitors pass high frequencies and block low frequencies.

Inductors block high frequencies and pass low frequencies.

Combining a capacitor and inductor blocks high and low frequencies with a minimum effect on the middle frequency range.

The Volume Control: The volume control is a variable resistor, regulating the current flowing through the amplifier. More current flows with the volume turned up. Lowering the volume control makes the sound quieter as less current flows.

The volume control is also a gain control. Gain is an electrical term while volume is an acoustic term. Gain is dependant on frequency. The volume control may be a wheel, a screwdriver adjustable potentiometer, or a sensing surface requiring only a light touch.

Tone Control: Electronic controls change hearing instrument frequency response characteristics from the combined response of the microphone and receiver. Tone controls vary the relative strength of high and low frequencies using a filter network of resistances and capacitors in the amplifier circuit.

Dampers, horns, earmold cavities, etc. can also change the frequency response.

Two types of tone controls in common use are click stop labelled H1, H2, H3, etc, and potentiometers with a screwdriver adjustable continuously variable tone control.

High frequency emphasis is low frequency suppression: low frequency emphasis is high frequency suppression.

The choice of receiver or microphone can also control frequency response. Mechanical controls, like dampers or foam, restrict the microphone or receiver openings and affect frequency response.

Passive Tone Controls are cost effective and use limited space. A hearing instrument with passive filtering usually routes the signal through a capacitor filter located between amplifier stages.

Active Tone Controls permit a broader fitting range, using feedback and phase relationships, and several transistor stages controlled by a program switch.

Output Controls: Output controls are either potentiometers or click switches. The labelling of the pots gives some clues to the type of circuit inside.

For example, if the range of the pot is from 119 dB to 138 dB, we know we are controlling the output. As the output is above 125 dB, we probably have a push-pull Class B linear circuit. We either have peak clipping or output compression.

Noise Switch: A noise switch or noise filter suppresses low frequencies, acting much like a patient adjustable tone control. The low frequency suppression reduces the masking effect of low frequency background noise, but allows the patient the advantage of the lower frequencies in quiet situations.

Telecoil: The telecoil is a magnetic induction coil that looks like a rod with copper wire wrapped around it. The telecoil responds to magnetic leakage from telephone receivers. It is also useful in classrooms, theatres, etc., anywhere with induction loop systems. With a separate induction coil, boot, or neck loop, you can couple directly to a radio, TV, or assistive listening device.

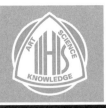
TEST INSTRUCTIONS

After you have finished reading this lesson, carefully study the selections from the **Required Reading.**

Then, look over the lesson once more to impress the important points on your memory.

When you are sure you know the lesson thoroughly, use the answer sheet in the back of the manual that corresponds to this lesson.

IMPORTANT: Place your student number on the answer sheets. Your student number appears on the inside front cover of the manual. **It must appear on your answer sheets in order for you to get credit for completion of the lesson.**

Once the answer sheet is completed, tear it out and mail to: International Institute for Hearing Instruments Studies
16880 Middlebelt Road, Suite 4, Livonia, MI 48154-3367

REQUIRED READING FOR THIS LESSON

Pages 6-8, 48-60
Hearing Instrument Science and Fitting Practices (Second Edition)

TEST QUESTIONS

1. **Sound cannot travel through the following medium or mediums:**
   a. gas
   b. vacuum
   c. gas or solid
   d. solid or liquid

2. **Any complex sound can be broken down into individual frequencies by a technique known as:**
   a. standing wave analysis
   b. Fourier spectral analysis
   c. transverse wave energy analysis
   d. stable molecular movement analysis

3. **How many octaves occur from 125 Hz to 2000 Hz?**
   a. 7 octaves
   b. 5 octaves
   c. 4 octaves
   d. 3 octaves

4. **The quality or timbre of a sound is a property that depends on:**
   a. how many frequencies are in the complex sound
   b. the relative strength of each frequency
   c. the resonance of the sound cavities
   d. all of the above

5. **The speed of sound in air, in feet per second, is:**
   a. 340
   b. 960
   c. 1100
   d. 1500

6. **What does the term "67 dB" mean?**
   a. half the total range of intensities
   b. 67 dB of acoustic power
   c. sound pressure level of 67 dB
   d. it is meaningless without a reference level

7. **The decibel is:**
   a. an absolute value
   b. used only as a measure of hearing loss
   c. an absolute measure of sound loudness
   d. a ratio between two intensities

8. **The weakest sound normal human ears can hear in the most sensitive frequency range of the ear is an effective sound pressure of about:**
   a. .5 dB
   b. 0 dB
   c. 0.00002 dynes/cm^2
   d. 0.0002 dynes/cm^2

9. **A formant is:**
   a. a frequency region within a complex tone where certain harmonics have relatively large energy
   b. a graph showing the loudness and frequency of the components of a complex sound
   c. the relative strength of all frequencies in a complex sound
   d. a synonym for pure tones

10. **The normal human ear canal resonance is in the approximate range of:**
    a. 2500 - 8000 Hz
    b. 5000 - 6000 Hz
    c. 2500 - 4000 Hz
    d. 100 -1500 Hz

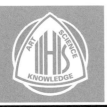
TEST INSTRUCTIONS

After you have finished reading this lesson, carefully study the selections from the **Required Reading.**

Then, look over the lesson once more to impress the important points on your memory.

When you are sure you know the lesson thoroughly, use the answer sheet in the back of the manual that corresponds to this lesson.

IMPORTANT: Place your student number on the answer sheets. Your student number appears on the inside front cover of the manual. **It must appear on your answer sheets in order for you to get credit for completion of the lesson.**

Once the answer sheet is completed, tear it out and mail to: International Institute for Hearing Instruments Studies
16880 Middlebelt Road, Suite 4, Livonia, MI 48154-3367

REQUIRED READING FOR THIS LESSON

Pages 60-71, 161-166
Hearing Instrument Science and Fitting Practices (Second Edition)

TEST QUESTIONS

1. **The harmonics of speech reinforce some frequencies more than others.
    The reinforced frequencies are:**
    a. a result of the Lombard effect
    b. a result of the Stenger effect
    c. formants
    d. the fundamental frequency

2. **Vowels differ from consonants in that they:**
    a. use more open vocal cord voicing
    b. have more high frequency energy
    c. have less volume
    d. are of shorter duration

3. **When tilting the frequency response, the last number in a matrix, i.e. 110/37/15, means:**
    a. a 15 dB/octave rise
    b. parallel venting produces this rise
    c. the 15 dB difference occurs between 500 Hz and the first peak
    d. this is the amount of dB required to eliminate the occlusion effect

4. **The patient's MCL on a speech circuit of the audiometer is usually judged on:**
   a. the occlusion effect
   b. the volume at 1000 Hz
   c. the ear canal resonance
   d. the high frequency energy required for clear speech

5. **ANSI developed the Articulation Index (AI) to express:**
   a. speech power
   b. speech clarity
   c. speech voicing
   d. speech articulation

6. **'Positive reinforcement' involves:**
   a. praising the patient for each accomplishment
   b. using the 'speech envelope' to counsel clients
   c. power and clarity curves
   d. presenting a tone that is only inaudible without the instrument on

7. **Our quest of improving speech understanding begins by studying:**
   a. speech production
   b. vowel consonant similarities
   c. power vs intensity
   d. all of the above

8. **Most auditory systems follow a power law. This logarithmic concept is:**
   a. if we make a sound twice as intense, the sound is twice as loud
   b. a 6 dB increase in sound pressure doubles the loudness
   c. a 10 dB increase in sound pressure doubles the loudness
   d. a 10 dB increase in loudness doubles the sound pressure

9. **Sones compare:**
   a. loudness across frequencies
   b. loudness up frequency
   c. abnormal loudness growth
   d. loudness in critical bands

10. **Mels measure:**
    a. auditory fatigue
    b. equal loudness contours
    c. intensity
    d. pitch

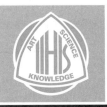
TEST INSTRUCTIONS

After you have finished reading this lesson, carefully study the selections from the **Required Reading.**

Then, look over the lesson once more to impress the important points on your memory.

When you are sure you know the lesson thoroughly, use the answer sheet in the back of the manual that corresponds to this lesson.

IMPORTANT: Place your student number on the answer sheets. Your student number appears on the inside front cover of the manual. **It must appear on your answer sheets in order for you to get credit for completion of the lesson.**

Once the answer sheet is completed, tear it out and mail to: International Institute for Hearing Instruments Studies
16880 Middlebelt Road, Suite 4, Livonia, MI 48154-3367

REQUIRED READING FOR THIS LESSON

Pages 128-131, 142-162, 304-317, 431-484, 804-810
Hearing Instrument Science and Fitting Practices (Second Edition)

TEST QUESTIONS

1. **Dexterity of a patient's fingers enter into the choice of instruments because of difficulty in:**
   a. inserting the earmold into the ear
   b. replacing the battery
   c. adjusting the volume or any of the controls of the hearing aid
   d. all of the above

2. **A bone conduction instrument should be used when:**
   a. a flat response is needed
   b. a monaural fitting is required
   c. pure tone testing indicates that bone conduction is worse than air conduction
   d. the patient has chronic otitis media

3. **A basic problem for clients with an asymmetrical hearing loss is:**
   a. discriminating speech from the side of the head with no usable hearing
   b. an inability to locate sound
   c. hearing in the presence of noise
   d. all of the above

4. **Pressure Measuring Instruments (PMI's) are:**
   a. built to the sound pressure standard of 20 micropascals
   b. no better for determining hearing aid needs than the speech audiometer
   c. usually unreliable for test re-test situations
   d. more complicated to operate than a speech audiometer

5. **Properly selected hearing instruments should allow:**
   a. the patient to wear an instrument at a comfortable loudness level
   b. improved communication ability of normal conversational speech in noise
   c. better hearing, aided, than unaided
   d. all of the above

6. **Slope of loss can determine a successful fitting. A most favorable slope is:**
   a. flat or gradually falling
   b. deep saucer shape
   c. sharp drop at a lower frequency
   d. irregular dips and peaks in thresholds

7. **Calculations of amplified sound to patients MCL do not include:**
   a. operating gain
   b. functional gain
   c. insertion gain
   d. reserve gain

8. **Calculating prescription formulas are compared to:**
   a. venting modifications
   b. specification sheets
   c. audiometric thresholds
   d. horn effects

9. **Some patients with binaural amplification can experience:**
   a. head shadow effect
   b. auditory deprivation
   c. degradation effect
   d. bilateral effect

10. **The following fitting requires amplification to two ears:**
    a. CROS
    b. BICROS
    c. binaural
    d. bone conduction

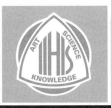
TEST INSTRUCTIONS

After you have finished reading this lesson, carefully study the selections from the **Required Reading.**

Then, look over the lesson once more to impress the important points on your memory.

When you are sure you know the lesson thoroughly, use the answer sheet in the back of the manual that corresponds to this lesson.

IMPORTANT: Place your student number on the answer sheets. Your student number appears on the inside front cover of the manual. **It must appear on your answer sheets in order for you to get credit for completion of the lesson.**

Once the answer sheet is completed, tear it out and mail to: International Institute for Hearing Instruments Studies
16880 Middlebelt Road, Suite 4, Livonia, MI 48154-3367

REQUIRED READING FOR THIS LESSON

Pages 311 - 317
Hearing Instrument Science and Fitting Practices (Second Edition)

TEST QUESTIONS

1. **Functional gain testing with CIC instruments is:**
    a. less time consuming than real-ear measurement with less test-retest variablility than sound field testing
    b. more time consuming than real-ear measurement and is difficult for the patient to understand
    c. simple for the patient to understand with less test-retest variablility than conventional sound field testing
    d. difficult for the patient to understand but is less time consuming than real-ear measurement testing

2. **With real ear measurement testing, which of the following is true:**
    a. placing the probe through the vent will appreciably change the frequency response
    b. the probe should be within 5 mm of the eardrum in order to avoid standing waves
    c. the probe should not extend beyond the tip of the hearing aid in order to avoid wave artifacts in the high frequency range
    d. the probe should extend at least 4 mm beyond the tip of the hearing aid

3. **The deeper microphone placement offers what advantage:**
    a. natural high frequency emphasis between 2700 and 4000 Hz
    b. reduction of the occlusion effect
    c. less gain requirements
    d. increased headroom wth undistorted output

4. **The deeper receiver placement offers what advantage:**
   a. natural high frequency emphasis between 2700 and 4000 Hz
   b. reduction of the occlusion effect
   c. decrease in wind noise
   d. increased headroom wth undistorted output

5. **CIC's offer a reduction in feedback for ALL but the following reasons:**
   a. less venting is required with CIC's
   b. increased headroom wth undistorted output
   c. CIC's are more tightly fitting
   d. less gain is required

6. **The Occlusion Effect is due to:**
   a. increase in bone-conduction sound for frequencies below 2000 Hz
   b. increase in bone-conduction sound for frequencies above 2000 Hz
   c. increase in air particle movement channeled out of the ear canal
   d. increase venting of the hearing aid mold

7. **When the wind is coming from directly ahead, wind noise is reduced in CIC's by the following amount:**
   a. 28 dB
   b. 27 dB
   c. 23 dB
   d. 7 dB SPL

8. **All but one of the following are considered possible disadvantages of CIC fittings:**
   a. introduction of programmable CIC's
   b. lack of a volume control
   c. cost
   d. higher return rate

9. **Earmold impressions for CIC's should:**
   a. extend to the second bend with medium viscosity, silicon material
   b. extend at least 2 mm beyond the second bend with light viscosity, silicon material
   c. extend to the second bend with light viscosity material using foam blocks
   d. extend at least 2 mm beyond the second bend using medium viscosity, silicon material

10. **With CIC fittings, which of the following frequency modifications should be made:**
    a. less low frequency amplification should be provided due to the small pinhole vent
    b. less high frequency amplification should be provided due to the deeper microphone placement
    c. deletion of automatic gain reduction due to the lack of volume control
    d. increased gain due to the difference in ear and 2 cc coupler gain differences

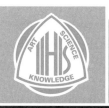

TEST INSTRUCTIONS

After you have finished reading this lesson, carefully study the selections from the **Required Reading.**

Then, look over the lesson once more to impress the important points on your memory.

When you are sure you know the lesson thoroughly, use the answer sheet in the back of the manual that corresponds to this lesson.

IMPORTANT: Place your student number on the answer sheets. Your student number appears on the inside front cover of the manual. **It must appear on your answer sheets in order for you to get credit for completion of the lesson.**

Once the answer sheet is completed, tear it out and mail to: International Institute for Hearing Instruments Studies
16880 Middlebelt Road, Suite 4, Livonia, MI 48154-3367

REQUIRED READING FOR THIS LESSON

Pages 238 - 239
Hearing Instrument Science and Fitting Practices (Second Edition)
Pages 1 - 10
Supplement – Digital Signal Processing for Hearing Aids

TEST QUESTIONS

1. **The Zeta Noise Blocker was:**
   a. an analog filter placed with a DSP hearing instrument
   b. a successful early attempt at digital noise reduction technology
   c. an example of a hybrid analog-digital hearing instrument
   d. none of the above

2. **The first commercially available Digital Signal Processing hearing instrument:**
   a. was developed by Audiotone
   b. included a body-worn electronic processor
   c. was introduced in 1986
   d. had better than average battery life

3. **A programmable hearing instrument with 4 channels and 1 memory could be considered a _____ programmable hearing instrument:**
   a. class 1
   b. class 2
   c. class 3
   d. class 4

4. **In digital signal processing, a set of mathematical steps involving multiplication, addition, and subtraction is referred to as:**
   a. an algorithm
   b. binary conversion
   c. analog to digital conversion
   d. imaging

5. **The number 512 would have a binary code of:**
   a. 100000101
   b. 1000000000
   c. 100000000
   d. 1111111111

6. **The sampling rate:**
   a. refers to how often the waveform amplitude is measured
   b. has a direct bearing on the frequency bandwidth of the hearing instrument
   c. must be at least twice as fast as the highest desired frequency
   d. all of the above

7. **Quantization is related to:**
   a. Aliasing
   b. Nyquist Theory
   c. number of bits
   d. all of the above

8. **The number of bits impact the:**
   a. dynamic range of the hearing instrument
   b. range of the hearing instrument transducers
   c. frequency resolution of the hearing instrument
   d. digital to analog conversion

9. **Imaging occurs during the:**
   a. analog to digital conversion stage
   b. signal processing stage
   c. digital to analog conversion stage
   d. receiver conversion of the electrical signal to an acoustic signal

10. **Which of the following is not an advantage attributable to digital signal processing in hearing instruments:**
    a. ability to use more channels for different types of signal processing
    b. implementation of noise reduction and speech enhancement features
    c. use of active filters for frequency response shaping
    d. all of the above are advantages attributable to digital signal processing

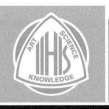
TEST INSTRUCTIONS

After you have finished reading this lesson, carefully study the selections from the **Required Reading.**

Then, look over the lesson once more to impress the important points on your memory.

When you are sure you know the lesson thoroughly, use the answer sheet in the back of the manual that corresponds to this lesson.

IMPORTANT: Place your student number on the answer sheets. Your student number appears on the inside front cover of the manual. **It must appear on your answer sheets in order for you to get credit for completion of the lesson.**

Once the answer sheet is completed, tear it out and mail to: International Institute for Hearing Instruments Studies
16880 Middlebelt Road, Suite 4, Livonia, MI 48154-3367

REQUIRED READING FOR THIS LESSON

(no required reading for this lesson)

TEST QUESTIONS

1. **One of the following does NOT apply to SIE-O fitted hearing aids:**
   a. Phase issues are eliminated
   b. The occlusion effect is minimized
   c. The speaker uses a soft silicone dome or molded, vented acrylic tip to secure the speaker in the ear canal
   d. Allows for more gain than does a SIA instrument

2. **Which statement is correct relative to the comparison between the SIE-O and SIE-S hearing instrument styles?**
   a. They provide the same overall performance
   b. The SIE-O provides greater acoustic advantages than does the SIE-S
   c. The SIE-S provides greater acoustic advantages than does the SIE-O
   d. Neither eliminates the occlusion effect because the speaker is placed in the ear canal

3. **SIA hearing aids are designed primarily to:**
   a. Reduce occlusion and the occlusion effect
   b. Provide for extended high-frequency amplification
   c. Provide maximum gain without acoustic feedback
   d. Avoid phase problems

4. **SIA open-fit hearing aid applicable gains, without feedback cancellation, shows that the maximum stable gain before feedback to be closest to:**
   a. 10 dB
   b. 20 dB
   c. 30 dB
   d. 40 dB

5. **The Vent as a two-channel device, is identified with:**
   a. A two-channel hearing aid in which one channel is programmed for the vent, and the other channel for the frequency response of the aid
   b. SIE-S hearing aids
   c. Any open fit or vented hearing aid
   d. Improved acoustic performance

6. **Small diameter tubing of SIA hearing aids has the effect of:**
   a. Providing greater high-frequency amplification
   b. Providing greater low-frequency amplification
   c. Providing the same gain as larger diameter tubing
   d. Reducing the high-frequency gain

7. **With SIE-S hearing aids:**
   a. The only signal is from the hearing aid and phase effects from a vent are not an issue
   b. Acoustic feedback can be managed only by use of feedback compression circuitry
   c. The occlusion effect is reduced/eliminated with the use of a vented earpiece
   d. Sealing the canal destroys overall acoustic performance

8. **Evidence suggests that the practical, maximum stable high-frequency gain of an open-fit device, when feedback cancellation is activated, is closest to:**
   a. 20 dB
   b. 25 dB
   c. 30 dB
   d. 35 dB

9. **Performance verification of SIA, SIE-O, and SIE-S hearing aid fittings is best made by:**
   a. Checking the programming software
   b. Real-ear probe microphone measurements
   c. Obtaining performance comments from the patient
   d. 2-cc coupler measurements

10. **One of the following is NOT a listed advantage of both the SIA and SIE hearing aid fittings:**
    a. Cosmetic improvement, rendering the instrument essentially "invisible" when worn
    b. Improved efficiency in the dispensing office
    c. Emphasis on earmold mechanics rather than on electroacoustics
    d. Same-session fit with patient having an opportunity to experience immediately the final fit (cosmetics, sound, comfort)

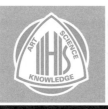

TEST INSTRUCTIONS

After you have finished reading this lesson, carefully study the selections from the **Required Reading.**

Then, look over the lesson once more to impress the important points on your memory.

When you are sure you know the lesson thoroughly, use the answer sheet in the back of the manual that corresponds to this lesson.

IMPORTANT: Place your student number on the answer sheets. Your student number appears on the inside front cover of the manual. **It must appear on your answer sheets in order for you to get credit for completion of the lesson.**

Once the answer sheet is completed, tear it out and mail to: International Institute for Hearing Instruments Studies
16880 Middlebelt Road, Suite 4, Livonia, MI 48154-3367

REQUIRED READING FOR THIS LESSON

Pages 237-244
Hearing Instrument Science and Fitting Practices (Second Edition)

TEST QUESTIONS

1. **When you cup your hand behind the ear, sound:**
   a. increases by 10-15 dB
   b. increases by 8-10 dB
   c. increases by 5-8 dB
   d. does not actually increase

2. **The first patent for a telephone type hearing instrument was in:**
   a. 1892
   b. 1903
   c. 1923
   d. 1930

3. **The first electric hearing instrument:**
   a. collected and amplified sound
   b. was used by Beethoven
   c. required vacuum tubes
   d. used a bone conduction device

4. **The carbon granule microphone:**
   a. was invented by Alexander Graham Bell in 1876
   b. caused static and fading with body movement
   c. became commercially available in the 1950's
   d. used a filament that generates heat

5. **Desk and suitcase sized hearing instruments, popular in the 1920's, had more gain and clarity because of:**
   a. the transistor
   b. carbon granule microphones
   c. magnetic earphones
   d. vacuum tube amplifiers

6. **Wearable instruments were a result of:**
   a. the arrival of the transistor
   b. the miniature vacuum tube
   c. the piezo-electrical microphone
   d. the magnetic microphone

7. **Crystal microphones and receivers:**
   a. work well in high temperatures
   b. use a filament that generates heat
   c. are very fragile
   d. couldn't withstand dry conditions

8. **A FET changed the high impedance problems of the:**
   a. magnetic microphone
   b. ceramic microphone
   c. carbon granule microphone
   d. electret microphone

9. **Magnetic microphones:**
   a. have high impedance
   b. have a good frequency response in the speech range
   c. have a poor response in the extreme highs and lows
   d. replaced the carbon microphones

10. **The miniature vacuum tube was introduced in about:**
    a. 1908
    b. 1920
    c. 1938
    d. 1948

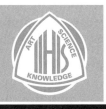
TEST INSTRUCTIONS

After you have finished reading this lesson, carefully study the selections from the **Required Reading.**

Then, look over the lesson once more to impress the important points on your memory.

When you are sure you know the lesson thoroughly, use the answer sheet in the back of the manual that corresponds to this lesson.

IMPORTANT: Place your student number on the answer sheets. Your student number appears on the inside front cover of the manual. **It must appear on your answer sheets in order for you to get credit for completion of the lesson.**

Once the answer sheet is completed, tear it out and mail to: International Institute for Hearing Instruments Studies
16880 Middlebelt Road, Suite 4, Livonia, MI 48154-3367

REQUIRED READING FOR THIS LESSON

Pages 237-245
Hearing Instrument Science and Fitting Practices (Second Edition)

TEST QUESTIONS

1. **The three major concepts in the use of electricity are:**
   a. current, voltage and resistance
   b. current, sound pressure and resistance
   c. current, power and resistance
   d. power, voltage and battery drain

2. **A capacitor:**
   a. passes the low frequencies and blocks the high frequencies
   b. blocks the low frequencies and passes the high frequencies
   c. passes both low and high frequencies
   d. blocks both low and high frequencies

3. **A resistor:**
   a. restricts low frequencies
   b. restricts high frequencies
   c. restricts the flow of electrons
   d. reverses the flow of electrons

4. **"Energy cannot be created or destroyed" is:**
   a. Ohm's law
   b. the law of conservation of energy
   c. the law of electricity
   d. the law of resistance

5. **The following is not a transducer:**
   a. receiver
   b. microphone
   c. volume control
   d. telephone coil

6. **Electrical energy uses the atom. Atoms:**
   a. are electrically neutral
   b. are electrically negative
   c. are electrically positive
   d. orbit around electrons

7. **Part of the basic law of electrical energy is:**
   a. protons repel neutrons
   b. protons repel electrons
   c. protons attract electrons
   d. electrons attract protons

8. **To produce current:**
   a. protons move from atom to atom
   b. atoms move from proton to electron
   c. electrons move from atom to atom
   d. electrons move from neutron to neutron

9. **A greater flow of current produces:**
   a. less battery gain
   b. more volume
   c. more timbre
   d. less intensity

10. **Semi-conductors act like a conductor with the application of:**
   a. heat, light or an electric field
   b. copper, gold or silver
   c. antimony, phosphorus or arsenic
   d. boron, aluminum or gallium

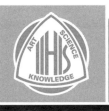
TEST INSTRUCTIONS

After you have finished reading this lesson, carefully study the selections from the **Required Reading.**

Then, look over the lesson once more to impress the important points on your memory.

When you are sure you know the lesson thoroughly, use the answer sheet in the back of the manual that corresponds to this lesson.

IMPORTANT: Place your student number on the answer sheets. Your student number appears on the inside front cover of the manual. **It must appear on your answer sheets in order for you to get credit for completion of the lesson.**

Once the answer sheet is completed, tear it out and mail to: International Institute for Hearing Instruments Studies
16880 Middlebelt Road, Suite 4, Livonia, MI 48154-3367

REQUIRED READING FOR THIS LESSON

Pages 245-304
Hearing Instrument Science and Fitting Practices (Second Edition)

TEST QUESTIONS

1. **The function of a microphone is to:**
   a. amplify the acoustic signal
   b. pick up electro-magnetic signals
   c. convert electrical energy into acoustic energy
   d. convert acoustic energy into electrical energy

2. **Coupling in a hearing instrument refers to connecting:**
   a. the microphone to the amplifier
   b. the diaphragm of the microphone to the electro-magnet
   c. one stage of an amplifier to the next
   d. solid state materials to create a junction

3. **The 'T' position on a hearing aid switch can be used to:**
   a. amplify a telephone conversation
   b. couple a hearing aid into a loop inductor system
   c. couple directly into the audio of a radio or TV set with a separate induction coil
   d. all of the above

4. **The following components can change or modify the frequency response of a hearing instrument:**
   a. a microphone
   b. a volume control
   c. an output potentiometer
   d. an 'off' switch

5. **The following is a transducer:**
   a. electret microphone
   b. amplifier
   c. integrated circuit
   d. volume control

6. **Amplifiers:**
   a. shape the frequency response for the microphone
   b. generate distortion
   c. replaced dozens of transistors
   d. are always linear

7. **A linear amplifier has a 1:1 relationship. This means that if you rotate the volume control on a linear aid, you change:**
   a. the input only
   b. the kneepoint only
   c. the output only
   d. the gain and the output

8. **Hard peak clipping occurs in a:**
   a. class A amplifier
   b. class B amplifier
   c. push-pull circuit
   d. compression amplifier

9. **Peak rounding:**
   a. is instantaneous
   b. is linear
   c. causes harmonic distortion above the knee
   d. uses a feedback loop before the volume control

10. **There are two types of compression – input and output. The difference is:**
    a. with input compression, you can only control the output
    b. with output compression, you can only control the input
    c. one uses attack time, the other, release time
    d. the placement of the feedback loop

INTERNATIONAL INSTITUTE FOR HEARING INSTRUMENTS STUDIES

DISTANCE LEARNING for Professionals in HEARING HEALTH SCIENCES

IIHIS

Unit IV - Hearing Instrument Fitting

CONTENTS

Lessons contained in Unit IV describe ANSI standards and tests; earmold techniques; fitting and verification; follow-up care; maintenance, modifications and repair, and real-ear measurements.

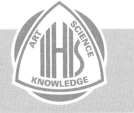

Published by
International Institute for Hearing Instruments Studies
Educational Division of International Hearing Society

INTERNATIONAL
INSTITUTE
FOR
HEARING
INSTRUMENTS
STUDIES

DISTANCE LEARNING
for Professionals in
HEARING HEALTH SCIENCES

ANSI STANDARDS

LESSON 24

Hearing instruments differ in both internal design and outer appearance or cosmetic appeal. Comparing one hearing instrument to another requires us to use the same measurements and parameters for each model. Then, we can determine if one instrument has an advantage over another for a particular patient, situation, or type of hearing loss. Each test must measure in exactly the same way, or comparisons are not possible.

The American National Standards Institute (ANSI) set standards for air conduction hearing instruments on how to measure performance, and what performances to measure. The ANSI standard, S3.22 - 1987, Specification of Hearing Instrument Characteristics, is in use today.

Each manufacturer uses this standard for measurement. The manufacturer also conducts measurements that demonstrate or reinforce a particular hearing instrument feature not covered by ANSI Standards, or uses measurements they want to become a future standard. We can compare different hearing instruments freely only when we measure each instrument using the same criteria, ANSI Standards.

The test equipment in common use for the measurement of hearing instruments is a hearing instrument analyzer system.

COUPLERS

The approximate volume of an average ear canal is 4 cc (cubic centimeters, also written cm^3). Consider that a solid earmold uses about half the volume of the canal, or 2 cc, leaving a remaining space of 2 cc. Hearing instrument measurements use a coupler connection allowing for the other half of the canal volume not used by the earmold or instrument itself. These couplers are 2 cc couplers. There are two types.

All in-the-ear and canal instruments use an HA 1 coupler. An HA 2 coupler connects behind-the-ear and pocket models. A measurement microphone fits into either coupler during testing. Fun-tack, silly putty or modelling clay seals the sound bore of the hearing instrument to the coupler.

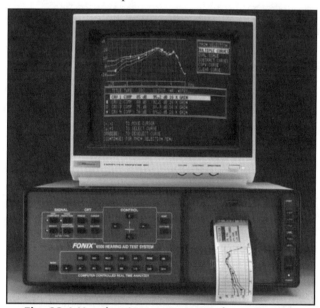

**Fig. 23-1 Hearing Instrument Analyzer System
(courtesy of Frye Electronics, Inc.)**

Figure 23-1 shows a computer screen readout above a panel with push button controls for selecting different tests. One of the buttons, ANSI, automatically runs the standard tests, but pauses in testing for you to reduce the volume of the hearing instrument to reference test position.

DEFINITIONS

Reference Sound Pressure Level: All sound pressure levels refer to 20 micro Pascals, which is the same as 0.0002 dynes/cm^2.

Input Sound Pressure Level: The input sound pressure level is the SPL **at the microphone opening of the**

hearing instrument for all nondirectional hearing instruments. The input SPL for directional hearing instruments is the SPL in a progressive sound field adjacent to the microphone openings of the hearing instrument.

Acoustic Gain: Acoustic gain is the difference between the output SPL and the input SPL in the 2 cc coupler.

Gain Control: Gain control is a user operated control for adjusting gain, the volume wheel.

AGC Control: An AGC control is any control that affects the steady state operation of the AGC function, excluding the user operated gain control, any tone control, or a peak clipping control.

Automatic Gain Control Hearing Instrument (AGC): An automatic gain control hearing instrument that incorporates a means other than peak clipping. The automatic control of gain is the input signal. The abbreviation for automatic gain control is AGC.

AGC Knee-Point: The knee-point on the input-output curve of an AGC hearing instrument is where the curve first departs from linear by 2 dB at input levels below the compression or limiting portion of the curve.

Directional Hearing instrument: A hearing instrument with microphone sensitivity dependent on the direction of sound, when measured under free-field conditions, is a directional hearing instrument.

ANSI TESTS

Using Sample Hearing Instrument Analyzer Graphs

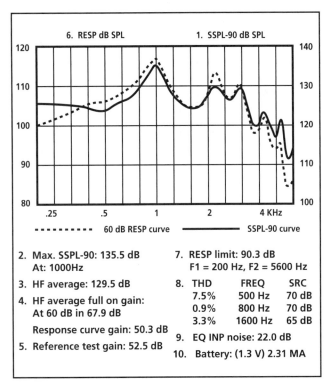

2. Max. SSPL-90: 135.5 dB
   At: 1000Hz
3. HF average: 129.5 dB
4. HF average full on gain:
   At 60 dB in 67.9 dB
   Response curve gain: 50.3 dB
5. Reference test gain: 52.5 dB

7. RESP limit: 90.3 dB
   F1 = 200 Hz, F2 = 5600 Hz

8. THD   FREQ   SRC
   7.5%   500 Hz   70 dB
   0.9%   800 Hz   70 dB
   3.3%   1600 Hz   65 dB

9. EQ INP noise: 22.0 dB
10. Battery: (1.3 V) 2.31 MA

Fig. 23-2 Linear Instrument

These graphs print in a continuous strip. They are only broken and divided for your comparison. Note the response graph uses the left column of numbers and the SSPL 90 graph reads from the right hand side.

1.	SSPL90
2.	Max SSPL90 @ ___ Hz
3.	HF Avg SSPL90
4.	HF AVG Full on gain
5.	Reference Test Gain
6.	Frequency Response curve
7.	Frequency range
8.	Total Harmonic Distortion
9.	Eq. Input Noise
10.	Battery Current Drain

Saturation Sound Pressure Level for 90 dB Input Sound Pressure Level (SSPL 90): The abbreviation for Saturation Sound Pressure Level for 90 dB is SSPL 90.

With the volume control set at maximum, **90 dB constant input tones across frequencies** force the hearing instrument to saturate. An SSPL 90 curve graphically displays the loudest sounds the hearing instrument can produce at every frequency over the range 200-5000 Hz.

This figure relates directly to UCL measurements, and is the first number in a matrix for ITE and canal orders, i.e. 114/42/15, (MPO/gain/slope).

High-Frequency Average Saturation Sound Pressure Level (HFA SSPL 90): High frequency average saturation sound pressure level is the **average of the SSPL90 values at 1000 Hz, 1600 Hz, and 2500 Hz,** abbreviated HFA-SSPL90.

Full-on Gain: Full on gain (FOG) is the acoustic gain the hearing instrument produces with a **sinusoidal 60 dB input** when the **volume control is full-on. Use a 50 dB SPL input for AGC instruments.**

Full-on gain is the middle number for ordering an ITE or canal with a matrix. The last number in the matrix is the rise, in dB, between 500 Hz and the first peak, i.e., **114/42/15.**

High-Frequency Average (HFA) Full-on Gain: High Frequency Average full on gain is an **average of the full-on gain values at 1000 Hz, 1600 Hz and 2500 Hz.**

Special Purpose Hearing Instrument (SPA): A special purpose hearing instrument is an instrument whose full-on gain at 1000, or at 1600 Hz or at 2500 Hz is less than the maximum full-on gain minus 15 dB. Extremely high frequency emphasis instruments fall into this category. You may have no gain at 1000 or 1600 Hz.

Reference Test Position (RTP): A linear hearing instrument would be in saturation with the volume control set at full on. To avoid saturation of the instrument and obtain a frequency response at a position closer to a user level for speech, turn the volume control down.

Since average speech is 65 dB SPL with a ± 12 dB variation in the intensity of phonemes, the average conversational maximum speech intensity would be 65 + 12 = 77 dB. Tests on the hearing instrument at this volume control setting allow the instrument to function with distortion free speech. **HFA SSPL 90 - 17 dB** is reference test position.

Your patient should wear the instrument at or below RTP, so the range of speech does not saturate the hearing instrument.

Reference Test Gain: Reference test gain position differs from reference test position **only by the 60 dB SPL input. Frequency response graphs include the 60 dB input SPL.** The volume wheel is at the same point. Reference Test Gain is HFA SSPL 90 - 17 - 60 input, or **HFA SSPL 90 - 77.** Reference test gain is the difference between output and input levels.

Frequency Response Curve: With the **volume control in reference test position and an input SPL of 60 dB,** run the frequency response curve. A frequency response curve includes the input sound pressure level of 60 dB SPL. **AGC hearing instruments require** full-on volume control and an input sound pressure level of 50 dB SPL.

Frequency Range: Determine the frequency range from the **frequency response curve** by finding the **average of 1000 Hz, 1600 Hz and 2500 Hz. Subtract 20 dB. Draw a horizontal line** parallel to the frequency axis at the reduced level. This is the frequency range line. The lowest frequency where your range line intersects the frequency response curve on the **left is F1.** The low-frequency limit is F1 or 200 Hz, whichever is higher. The **highest frequency, F2,** is where the frequency range line intersects the frequency response curve on the right. The high-frequency limit is the lower of F2 or 5000 Hz.

Harmonic Distortion: Harmonic distortion (HD) occurs when new frequencies generated are harmonics of the original input signal. A 400 Hz tone has harmonics at 800, 1200, 1600, etc. With the **gain control in the RTP,** measure harmonic distortion with a **70 dB input sound pressure level at 500 Hz, 800 Hz; 65 dB SPL input level at 1600 Hz.** Measure and record total harmonic distortion (THD) for each of the three frequencies.

Equivalent Input Noise Level (Ln): Random noise distortion occurs at each amplifier stage. The first amplifier is the most critical, because each succeeding stage amplifies the noise along with the desired signal. ANSI Standards measure Equivalent Input Noise Level with the **volume control at RTP.** Determine the average coupler SPL's at **1000, 1600 and 2500 Hz with a 60 dB SPL input. Remove the 60 dB SPL input** signal and record the sound pressure level in the coupler caused by inherent noise.

Battery Current: Measure battery current with a pure-tone **1000 Hz 65 dB input signal and the hearing instrument at RTP.**

The following tests apply to AGC instruments.

Input-Output characteristics: Using a pure tone frequency of **2000 Hz,** measure the coupler SPL for input **SPL's from 50 to 90 dB in 10 dB steps.** The measured curve at 50 and 90 dB input SPL must not differ in output SPL by more than ±5 dB from manufacturer's specs.

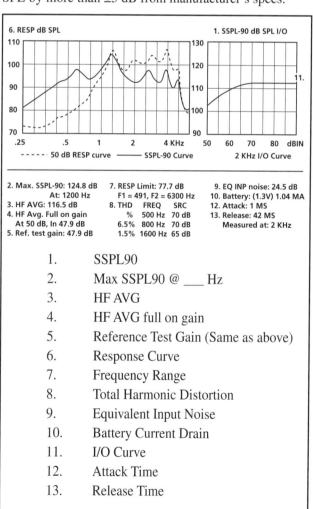

2. Max. SSPL-90: 124.8 dB	7. RESP Limit: 77.7 dB	9. EQ INP noise: 24.5 dB
At: 1200 Hz	F1 = 491, F2 = 6300 Hz	10. Battery: (1.3V) 1.04 MA
3. HF AVG: 116.5 dB	8. THD FREQ SRC	12. Attack: 1 MS
4. HF Avg. Full on gain	% 500 Hz 70 dB	13. Release: 42 MS
At 50 dB, In 47.9 dB	6.5% 800 Hz 70 dB	Measured at: 2 KHz
5. Ref. test gain: 47.9 dB	1.5% 1600 Hz 65 dB	

1. SSPL90
2. Max SSPL90 @ ___ Hz
3. HF AVG
4. HF AVG full on gain
5. Reference Test Gain (Same as above)
6. Response Curve
7. Frequency Range
8. Total Harmonic Distortion
9. Equivalent Input Noise
10. Battery Current Drain
11. I/O Curve
12. Attack Time
13. Release Time

Fig. 23-3
AGC Instruments

Dynamic AGC Characteristics

With the **gain control full-on, use a 2000 Hz pure-tone input signal** that alternates abruptly between **55 and 80 dB SPL.**

Attack time: the time between the abrupt increase from 55 to 80 dB and the point where the level has stabilized to within 2 dB of the steady value for the **80 dB input SPL.**

Release time: the interval between the abrupt drop from 80 to 55 dB and the point where the signal has stabilized to within 2 dB of the steady state value for the **55 dB input SPL.**

No matter what type of hearing instrument your patient wears, some form of earmold transmits the amplified sound from the hearing instrument to the eardrum. An earmold is an acoustic coupler. The tiniest canal instrument has characteristics in common with the largest earmold used with a behind-the-ear model.

Any hearing instrument fitting has basic requirements, whether the instrument is a molded impression of the ear, or attaches to the molded impression. It must:

1. Be aesthetically acceptable to the patient.

2. Be comfortable to wear for extended periods of time.

3. Maintain or enhance the frequency response and output of the hearing instrument circuitry.

Learning what an earmold can do is much easier if we realize there are two important parts - outer appearance, and canal acoustics.

OUTER APPEARANCE

In 1970, the National Association of Earmold Labs (N.A.E.L.) created standardized names for earmold physical styles. This list has not been revised, although earmold labs differ in their name for a particular earmold.

For instance, an earmold that fills the entire concha bowl and canal portion is a **shell** earmold. A shell earmold has tubing in the sound bore. Because material seals the canal and outer ear, these earmolds suit severe-to-profound losses. If you only fill the bottom half of the ear, then you have a **half-shell.**

If you wish to connect this type of earmold to a body-worn hearing instrument, it becomes a **receiver, or regular, or standard** earmold with metal or vinyl receiver clip rings.

One of the most popular styles of earmold is **skeleton.** Also known as **phantom,** or **silhouette,** this earmold outlines the rim of the outer ear while effectively sealing the canal, fitting a moderate-to-moderately severe loss. A earmold with less outer rim is **3/4 skeleton,** or **1/2 skeleton** (Semi-skeleton).

Removing the top half of a skeleton leaves a canal lock. Remove the lock for a **canal.** As we cut away the outer parts of the earmold, acoustic leakage can occur, causing feedback.

Canal Acoustics: Acoustic Compliance occurs when air is enclosed in an earmold with rigid walls. The sound follows the restricted path the earmold provides. Compliance partially exists in the ear canal, but not at all at the eardrum, which moves freely in and out with pressure changes. Highly compliant earmolds aid the transmission of high frequency sounds.

The Horn Effect: When the volume of air increases by 'belling' a canal or shortening a earmold, compliance increases. We can use special tubing that flares or 'bells' in 'steps', like a Libby Horn or Bakke Horn, or we can flare or step the sound bore. We can 'scoop out' the whole canal. Earmold labs call this adjustment a sound separator **or acoustic modifier.** All of these canal changes produce varying degrees of high frequency emphasis, increase compliance, and create an **acoustic transformer.**

Ear Canal Resonance: Milder losses require less material in the aperture and intertragal notch area, retaining **natural ear canal resonance. Free field** earmolds like **non-occluding free field, 2 HF, 2 HF Extended, and Janssen** earmolds have little or no material in the intertragal notch, but, being so open, are prone to feedback above 25 - 30 dB gain.

Venting: Any earmold occludes when no outside air enters directly into the canal, or becomes non-occluding with a parallel vent. A large parallel vent has the greatest effect on frequency response of any modification.

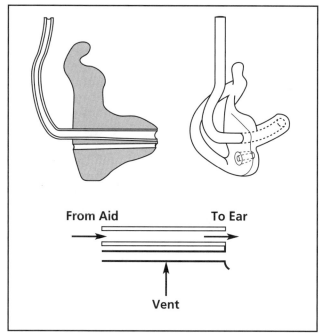

Fig. 24-1 Parallel Vent

A parallel vent opens up the canal on a shell, skeleton, or canal earmold, creating a non-occluding earmold. More and more ear canal resonance naturally occurs, depending on the size of the vent. Low frequencies bleed off through this opening, emphasizing higher frequencies, and affecting both gain and output by a few dB.

Acoustic inertance occurs when a volume of air oscillates without compressing to any significant extent, as in tubing, or a 'bore' at a vent.

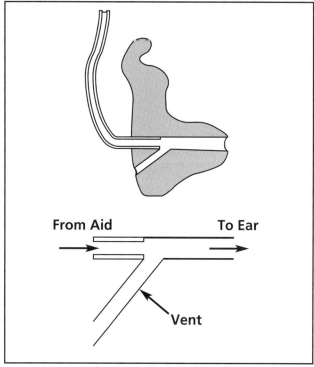

Fig. 24-2 Diagonal Vent

An angle, or diagonal vent from the intertragal notch into the 'sound bore' bleeds off only extreme lows. The diameter and length of the vent determine the acoustic effects. Tiny vent channels provide pressure relief without reducing gain or output. Sometimes more than one vent is necessary.

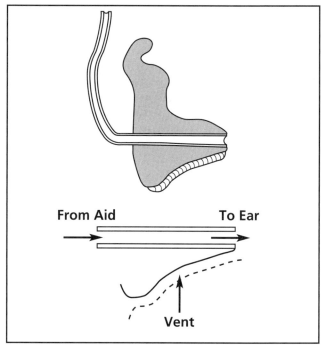

Fig. 24-3 External Vent

An external vent reduces fullness or occlusion, rather than fulfilling an acoustic modification. It is more practical to drill a vent on an ordinary earmold, or buff the entire surface of the canal of the earmold for comfort than to channel along the bottom of the earmold. External venting is most often used to solve a problem on an unvented ITE or canal instrument.

Continuous Flow Adapter (CFA) Earmolds combine a flare or 'stepped bore' with parallel vents (Bore 1, 2 and 3), open earmold fittings (Bore 4), diagonal vents (Bore 5) or unvented earmolds (Bore 4 and 5).

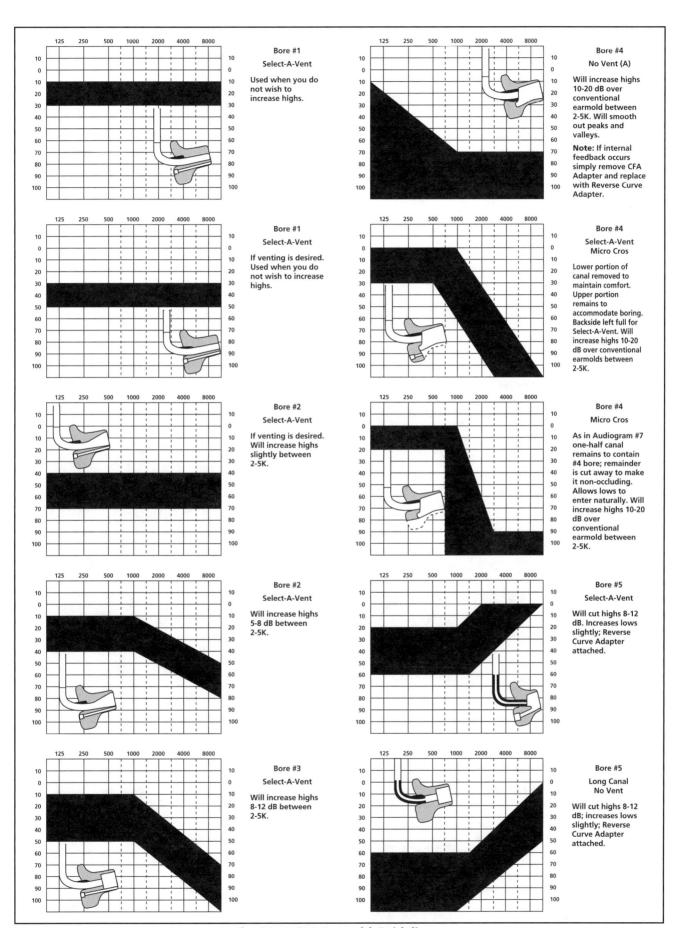

Fig. 24-4 CFA Earmold Guidelines

TUBING

The inside diameter (ID) of tubing and tubing length create significant variables in frequency response. The gain and output of any hearing instrument increases or decreases by changing tube diameter.

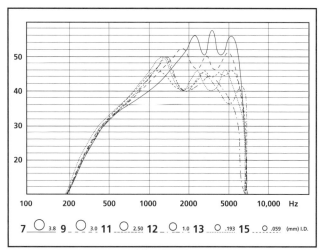

Fig. 24-5
Tubing Diameter

Use Heavy Wall (HW) tubing if feedback is a problem, or if the fitting is tubing only. Less sound leaks through the tubing wall. Sound cannot oscillate the heavier tubing as easily. Tube fittings are firmer and do not collapse when entering the aperture of the ear canal.

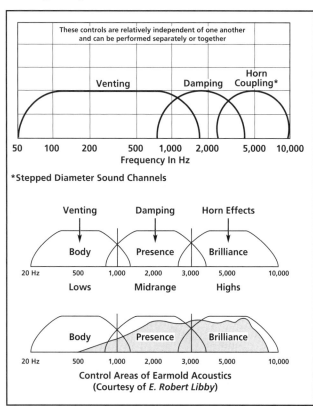

Fig. 24-6
Venting, Damping and Horn Effects

Acoustic control of earmolds falls into three independently variable areas. Earmold technology uses any or all of these areas on an earmold.

Acoustic impedance opposes or restricts the flow of sound through the system by either temporarily changing the acoustic flow with a resonating cavity, or dissipating energy.

Helmholtz resonance occurs in an earmold when a length of tubing is adjacent to a cavity with a volume of air enclosed in it.

FGM, and Macrae Anti-Feedback Earmolds use a resonating cavity.

DAMPERS OR FILTERS

Molds using dampers, filters, or lambs wool in the tubing, restrict the acoustic flow across frequencies, dissipating energy by frictional loss, and producing heat. Moisture builds up and condensation forms in the tubing.

The position of the filter or damper in the hearing instrument earhook, or in the earmold tubing, determines the frequency response change.

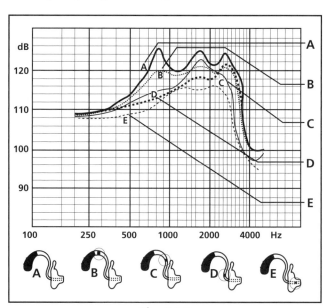

Fig. 24-7
Damper Positioning and Frequency Response Changes

MATERIAL OPTIONS

Any earmold can be extremely hard plastic or soft and pliable, or a combination of a hard earmold with a soft canal tip. Deciding factors in earmold materials are power level requirements, patient dexterity, ear texture, allergy problems, and cosmetic appeal.

Lucite earmolds dominate for ease of modification, maintenance, durability, and cosmetic appeal. When allergy is a consideration, use **Polyethylene,** a semi-rigid white material, resembling paraffin wax. When power is a requirement, try **silicone. Soft materials** for earmolds use Poly Ethyl Methacrylate, a material that softens with body temperature. Add this material to the canal portion of a lucite earmold for high gain hearing instruments.

EARMOLD TECHNIQUES

Types of Impression Materials:

There are many different types of materials available for taking impressions. Most of these materials come in one of two basic types; a two part powder and liquid mix or a silicone based mix.

Powder and Liquid: This may come in large quantities, referred to as bulk, or in individual, pre measured, packages. The mixing is done at the time the impression is to be taken; using a mixing cup and spatula. Careful packaging of the finished impression is important to prevent distortion during shipping and handling.

Add the powder to liquid during mixing. First pour the liquid into the mixing cup, then add the powder. Moisten the powder, then stir vigorously. At first, the material looks like it is mixed with water. As you continue to stir, the mixture becomes creamy, like it is mixed with milk, and malleable. When the mixture reaches this stage it is ready to load into the syringe.

Silicone: Silicone comes in bulk, and resembles silly putty. It requires a hardening agent which may be in creamy form and mixed half and half, or in toothpaste tube form and added to the silicone putty. The putty and hardener is harder to mix in a cup than with the hands. You can knead the material, mixing it more evenly, using the palms. It should be all one color, not streaky, for best results. When the color is achieved, form a cone shaped mass and drop it into the syringe.

The newest silicone product comes in separate tubes and requires a gun. The material and hardener mixes itself as it proceeds through the disposable tip. The used tip remains on the gun until the next impression is required. When ready to take the next impression replace the used tip with a new tip. You must work slowly when using the gun to insure proper mixing of the material and hardener.

The quality of an earmold or hearing instrument case is directly related to the quality of the impression. It is better to re-do the impression as often as necessary for a perfect impression. Be very critical of your work. It is better to waste a few impressions to start with; the more impressions you take the better you will become.

Equipment and Materials:

To take the ear impression you will need the following equipment and materials:

1. Otoscope
2. Earlite
3. Cotton or foam dams
4. Impression material
5. Mixing cup
6. Spatula
7. Syringe

Optional Equipment
• Blunt ended tweezers
• Blunt nosed scissors

Steps To Taking An Impression:

One: Preparation for making the impression must include hygienic procedures that are strictly followed as a matter of routine. Thoroughly wash your hands with soap and warm water before and after making the ear impression. Clean the specula of the otoscope, ear-light tip, syringe, etc., with an antiseptic solution like Benzalkonium Chloride or a viricide solution. The items used for taking the impression should be stored dry, in sanitary glass containers or plastic bags.

Caution: Avoid using alcohol or other antiseptics injurious to plastics.

Two: Conduct a thorough otoscopic examination of the ear before taking the impression. An earlite is no substitute for an otoscopic examination and should not be used to examine the ear and ear canal. The earlite is used to place the cotton or foam dam properly in the ear canal, **NOT** to inspect the ear or ear canal. During the otoscopic examination check for the following:

1. Foreign objects in the ear canal.
2. Excessive wax in the ear canal which could distort the impression or cause feedback when the hearing instrument is put in place.
3. Abnormal growths in the ear or ear canal.
4. Any condition which is out of the ordinary.

If any of the above are found, stop and refer the patient to the appropriate medical professional. Do not continue with the impression.

5. Check the ear canal for size, this will determine how large a dam you will need to block the canal completely without distorting the canal.
6. Check which way the canal twists and bends. This gives you an idea of the direction to push the dam for insertion in the proper position.
7. Check for a possible prolapsed canal. When found, a larger than normal size dam is required.
8. Check for loose skin. Loose skin may require a tapering of the end of the earmold or hearing instrument to insure proper fitting.

9. Check for landmarks in the canal. Look for the second bend. This is where the final placement of the dam should be.

10. Look for any bumps, (moles, pimples, ridges) and hollows in the ear canal and circle them on the impression. In this way, the lab will not fill them in thinking they were just air bubbles or other irregularities.

Dam Placement:

Always use a cotton or foam dam the same size, or slightly larger than the second bend of the ear canal. This acts as a complete block of the canal, and it will not move when the impression material is forced against the dam. Without the dam packing or using a smaller dam, the material tapers in the canal, giving a false and smaller "picture" of the canal.

There are many prepackaged foam and cotton dams on the market. They come in a variety of sizes. There are times when you require a size that you don't have. In this case, use more than one whenever you are in doubt. Use several on post-surgical ears. It is not uncommon to use up to six or seven large dams on post-surgical ears. Five is common and three is average.

When a prolapsed canal is present, use a dam large enough to hold the canal open to a normal size.

Sometimes, when you require a very small block, it is better not to cut an existing block down to size — tie your own. If you need an extremely large dam, use cotton balls and dental floss to tie your own dams.

Place the dam in the opening of the ear canal with your fingers. While pulling up the back on the ear as you do for an otoscopic examination, use the earlite to slide the dam into the ear canal, up past the second bend. The earlite will allow you to see the penetration, the blockage of the canal, and be assured of its proper positioning at 90 degrees to the canal wall. Do not push the dam straight in with the earlite but rather gently push top and bottom, side-to-side and walk the dam into place slowly and gently.

If you are in doubt as to whether you have the proper positioning, there is another way to figure out the proper placement depth. After making an otoscopic inspection of the ear and locating the second bend, switch to the earlite. Before putting in the dam, turn on the earlite and insert the earlite tip in to the required depth. Hold the stem of the earlite so your fingers are flush with the rim of the ear. Withdraw the light. Mark the spot with your pen. Insert the dam. When your spot is again at the rim of the ear, you will be sure that the dam is in the proper position. The light from the tip shows you that the dam is in straight. The mark on the stem indicates the proper depth.

If the dam is in the canal, and you're not sure that it is in far enough, release your grip on the ear. Look again with your earlite, without touching the ear. With proper insertion, almost none of the dam is seen as it is around the corner of the second bend, out of sight.

Earmolds improve high frequency emphasis by increasing canal length into the isthmus of the canal, beyond the second bend.

Each time the length of the mold is increased by half the distance between the mold and the eardrum, intensity doubles… an increase of 6 dB. When the mold extends past the second bend, the occlusion effect is no longer a problem. The hearing instrument appears louder because the distance to the eardrum is shorter. Long canal technology is especially advantageous with moderate to severe losses as both frequency and intensity increase.

Syringe Method of Impression Taking:

The syringe method allows you to use the material in a softer state, and inject the material into the ear. This helps to eliminate the problem of distorting a soft or flexible ear. Obtain a softer texture by mixing the material for less time, not by using more liquid or less powder. Never change the recommended proportions of material.

Mix the impression material and place it into the barrel of the spatula. When taking impressions on children, be sure to use less material than you would with an adult. The additional weight of the material will distort the ear. Sometimes, it is easier to mix the normal amount of material.

Insert the plunger and force the material to within 1/8" of the end of the nozzle, to eliminate air pockets. If you think that the consistency is too loose, squeeze out about 1/4" while holding the tip horizontal. The impression material should hold its horizontal shape without drooping. If it droops, wait a few seconds and try again.

Pull the ear up and backward to straighten the canal. Place the tip of the nozzle 1/8" into the canal. Squeeze, forcing the material up to the dam, fill the canal, then release your grip on the ear. Let the ear return to its normal position. Keep the tip buried in the material as it flows out of the syringe. Back out, buried in the material, until the canal is full.

Remain buried in the material, and work your way up to the helix, at an angle, so air is not trapped at the helix tip. Back down, still buried and fill the concha bowl, covering the antihelix rim, intertragal notch and tragus. It is not necessary to touch the impression material at all.

When working with the heavier silicone, watch that the skin in the helix and tragus area does not move outward as you fill the ear. If either skin moves, gently massage it back into place while continuing to fill the ear.

If you remain buried in your impression material as you fill the ear, you will not have air pockets, cracks, lines or bubbles. Nor, will you have distorted the ear with any manual pressure.

Have your client open their mouth wide, close it and swallow, chew vigorously, and move the jaw from side to side, smile, and wiggle their ears if they can. You see lots of ear movement on some people when they go from serious to smiling. If you see this, have them repeat the serious to smiling action. Turn the head to both left and right as far as possible. This allows for normal movement of the canal tissue, and less likelihood of the finished earmold working our of the ear or whistling during normal activities.

Allow the impression material to set up for ten to twelve minutes before trying to remove it from the ear.

Feel the rim of the impression when you have finished filling the ear. You will notice that it feels very oily. (Powder and liquid only). When the material sets sufficiently for removal, the rim of the material will feel dry and sandy to a light touch.

Test silicone impressions with your fingernail. Your fingernail leaves a dent in the impression when you finish filling the ear. When the impression material sets properly, even heavy pressure with the fingernail leaves no mark.

When the impression has 'set-up' gently loosen the rim of the ear away from the impression. Holding the string from the dam and the bottom of the impression with the same hand, rock the impression with an upward and backward motion so you are pulling the canal portion out more than the helix. Removal is easier on sharp bend canals if the client opens their mouth. This is not usually necessary. Be very careful not to stretch or tear the canal on the impression. The dam remains attached to the finished ear impression.

Inspect the ear with an otoscope. No material should remain in the ear canal. There should be no marks from your installation of the dam.

INSPECTION of the IMPRESSION:

Inspect your impression for
1. A full canal, complete, with the second bend.
2. A full thickness of the canal aperture.

3. A full helix, complete with the curl.
4. A clearly shown tragus.
5. A complete bowl.

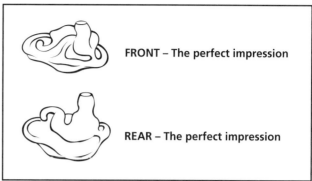

FRONT – The perfect impression

REAR – The perfect impression

Fig. 24-8 (Courtesy Hocks Laboratories, Inc.)

There should be no lumps, valleys, cracks or bubbles. These are caused by lifting the syringe out of the material. If there is a hollow anywhere on the impression, check the same spot in the ear for a bump that you may have missed. If you find a bump in the ear at that spot, circle the hollow in the impression. Make a note on the order form, so the area is not filled, or it will be uncomfortable for your patient. The texture of the hollow in the impression appears like the texture of the rest of the impression when a bump is present. An error in making the impression creates a shiny hole because the material only came in contact with the air.

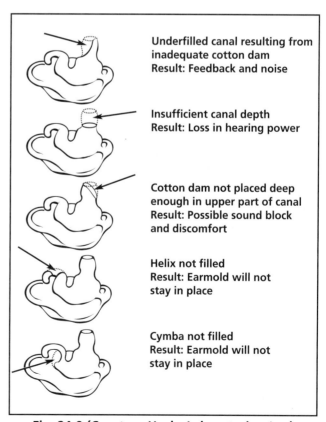

Underfilled canal resulting from inadequate cotton dam
Result: Feedback and noise

Insufficient canal depth
Result: Loss in hearing power

Cotton dam not placed deep enough in upper part of canal
Result: Possible sound block and discomfort

Helix not filled
Result: Earmold will not stay in place

Cymba not filled
Result: Earmold will not stay in place

Fig. 24-9 (Courtesy Hocks Laboratories, Inc.)

If the impression is defective or incomplete in any portion, make another immediately. Modify your procedures, as needed, to achieve a full and satisfactory impression.

There are three other methods used for the taking of impressions. They are the **Hand Pack Method,** the **Tamper Method,** and the **Gun Method.** These methods need to be mentioned but the most common method used today in the industry is the syringe method just described.

In the hand pack method the material is mixed with a spatula until the material begins to gather together and comes away from the sides of the bowl. Remove the material from the bowl. If it is tacky, knead or roll it in your hands until it stops adhering. Pinch off about one third of the material. Roll it into a carrot-like shape. Gently grasp and pull the pinna out and up from the head. This will open the canal, so a full, long impression is obtained. Direct the carrot-shaped material into the ear canal with the other hand. Press vigorously, at least five or six times, with the small finger.

Make sure that the material has reached the dam. The canal and part of the concha will be filled. Take the balance of the material, finish packing the concha, and work the material up into the helix. Make sure the helix is not 'closed off', creating an air pocket. If you do not have the ear satisfactorily packed by now, one more push is not going to do the job. At this stage of firmness, you may distort the ear. The

material has set up. When the material has been removed from the bowl, complete the packing of the ear within 30 seconds. More packing will distort the ear.

Be careful not to stretch a soft ear out of shape. Many earmold problems, caused by pressing to much material into a soft ear, result in over-sized, misshaped impressions.

The tamper method requires a tamper tool, which is a spatula, with a tamper at the top. Long strokes with the tool pack impression material deep in a small or narrow canal.

The gun method follows the syringe method, with one exception. **NEVER BURY THE TIP OF THE SYRINGE** or you will get little holes and creases all over the impression. Work very slowly, as this material has an extremely loose texture.

Glue powder and liquid impressions to the box, canal up. If the impression is not flat enough to glue, a razor blade cuts a smooth, flat surface. Drape order forms over the box, extending downward on the sides. The lid of the box holds the order forms in place. If you require pins to hold the canal upright, make the pins visible, and mark "PINS" IN BOLD LETTERS ON THE ORDER FORM.

Silicone impressions have a much better memory than powder and liquid impressions, retaining their shape during packaging and shipping, without fear of distortion.

Modification & Effect Chart

	Modification	Effect on Low Frequencies (Below 750 Hz)	Effect on Frequencies Between 750 and 1500Hz	Effect on Frequencies Between1500 and 3000 Hz	Effect on High Frequencies (Above 3000 Hz)
Tubing Diameter	Larger I.D. Tubings & Horn Tubing	Negligible	Moves peak to higher frequency	Increases height of peak and moves to higher frequency	Increases
	Smaller I.D. Tubing	May reduce below 1 KHz	Moves peak to lower frequency	Reduces height of peak and moves to lower frequency	Reduced by large decrease
Tubing Length	Longer Tubing	Increased	Moves peak to lower frequency	Moves peak to lower frequency	Negligible
	Shorter Tubing	Slight.y Decreases	Moves peak to higher frequency	Moves peak to higher frequency	Negligible
Length of Earmold Canal	Longer Earmold Canal	Increases level of response curve			
	Shorter Earmold Canal	Decreases level of response curve			
Bore Diameter	Larger Diameter Bore Through Earmold Canal*	Negligible	Moves peak to higher frequency	Moves peak to higher frequency	Increases
	Smaller Diameter Bore Through Earmold Canal*	Negligible	Moves peak to lower frequency	Moves peak to lower frequency	Decreases
Bore Length	Longer Bore Through Earmold Canal*	Slightly Increases	Moves peak to lower frequency	Moves peak to lower frequency	Decreases
	Shorter Bore Through Earmold Canal*	Slightly Decreases	Moves peak to higher frequency	Moves peak to higher frequency	Increases
Select-A-Vent	Very Small Vent (.031)**	Negligible	Negligible	Negligible	Negligible
	Small Vent (.042) **	Decreases	Negligible	Negligible	Negligible
	Medium Vent (.064) **	Decreases	Increases peak height	Negligible	Nebligible
	Large Vent (.089) **	Decreases	Increases peak height	Negligible	Negligible
Non-Occluding Mold	Non-Occluding Mold	Eliminates	Moves peak to higher frequency and increases height	Increases peak height	Negligible
Open Vent Mold	Open-Vented (High Frequency) Mold	Decreases	Reduces peak height	Negligible	Negligible
Filter Inserts	Filter Insert at Hearing Aid Nub	Negligible	Reduces peak height	Reduces peak height	Negligible
	Filter Insert At Earmold Tip	Slightly Decreases	Large Reduction	Large Reduction	Decreases

NOTE: Because of wide variation in earphone types and internal acoustical systems in hearing aids this chart must be considered as a guide for average conditions.

* Applies to earmolds for conventional earphones.

** Vents of short lengths are more effective in reducing low frequency response. Gain must be limited with larger size vents to avoid feedback.

Fig. 24-10
Earmold Modifications and Effects

THE FITTING

LESSON 26

The successfully fitting of a hearing instrument(s) depends on effectively teaching your patient how to operate and insert the instrument. However, instructions are not enough. You must guide and counsel on a continuing basis about what to expect and what **not** to expect from the new instrument. Your patient must feel that you are there to assist at all times.

A hearing instrument fitting occurs when the patient receives the hearing instrument, but must return for individual adjustments, verifications and check-ups. Any visit after the patient is fit with the instrument is Post Fitting Care. Any test, measurement, or exercise you give them to prove the success of the fitting is Fitting Verification. Fitting, verification and post fitting care are critical to successful use. The finest acoustic instrument in the world is worthless unless it satisfies the needs of the patient.

Residual hearing will be enhanced with the hearing instrument. A hearing instrument will not replace or restore hearing to normal. It may not even sound natural at first. It can help improve communication better provided both of you work together for the next few weeks. Encourage your patient to share information and experiences with family and friends to help make a smooth adjustment to the hearing instrument.

Show the patient the instrument and earmold, explain each part, the entire shape, the canal, the outer surface, the helix, how it sits in or on the ear, and what position it sits in. Use the wax pick (wax brush) to demonstrate cleaning, suggest a soft cloth to wipe the instrument or earmold.

Teach your patient how to insert and remove the instrument or earmold. Have the patient insert and remove an earmold several times before attaching the instrument. Demonstrate the controls on the hearing instrument. Show the patient both sides of the battery, how the difference between the plus and minus side can be felt, and how to insert and remove the battery.

Suggestions should be made to open the battery door at night. The battery itself does not need to be removed. Moisture can evaporate, the instrument cannot work, even if they forget to turn it off.

Insert the earmold in the ear again and place the behind-the-ear instrument on the ear. Measure the tubing to insure an overlap on the elbow of 1/8 to 1/4 inch then cut the tubing. Attach the earmold to the hearing instrument. Re-insert the earmold, place the hearing instrument behind the ear and CHECK THE FIT. It should sit comfortably on the top of the ear and rest along the back of the ear.

THE VOLUME CONTROL

Your instructions on adjusting the volume control are critical to the patient using the hearing instrument(s) effectively. The patient should expect a change in their voice.

Normal is a range. It is not an exact, precise spot on the volume control. Your patient wants to hear soft speakers and normal speakers. They want other clues in their speech. Are they speaking softly because they are embarrassed? Or shy? Or only want you to hear their secret?

VERIFY MCL and UCL

All your conversation with the patient helps to establish and approve of a comfortable listening level. Also check uncomfortable level. Rattle paper, make noises, use a noise tape while carrying on a conversation. If the patient cannot answer your questions in noise, make adjustments. You are checking overload.

TELEPHONE COIL

If the hearing instrument has an O-T-M setting, with the instrument in the T position, the patient cannot hear through the hearing instrument. The T position generally disconnects the microphone from the circuit, and connects the induction loop. Demonstrating the use of a telephone coil works better if you explain how it works first.

1. Switch from M to the T Position.

2. Turn the volume louder.

3. Hold the phone to the hearing instrument. When the hearing instrument is a BTE, hold the phone behind the ear, usually near the T switch.

4. An alternate use for the telecoil is as a coupler for assistive listening devices.

When switching from T to M, to avoid feedback, turn the volume control down.

HOW to ADJUST to YOUR HEARING INSTRUMENT

In your own words explain:

1. Adjusting to your new hearing instrument takes time and patience. Don't expect to learn everything the first day. Wear your instrument at home, listening to the sounds around you, even if there is no one to talk to. You'll be aware of sounds, like the tap dripping, the fridge clicking on or running, the little sounds you make as you move around. Each time you hear a sound, find out what it is. Then, when you hear it again, you'll recognize it, and it will bother you less and less. A hearing instrument does not amplify sounds unless it hears them.

2. Practice talking to just one person. Have the person sit six to eight feet away. This is an ideal distance to become confident with the adjustment of the volume at your comfortable level.

3. Suggest that your family and friends attract your attention before they speak to you. They raise their voices to you, and may need a gentle reminder to speak quietly or slowly.

4. Practice listening to the radio and TV with your hearing instrument on. You should find them much clearer without being loud.

5. As your hearing decreased, you found it more and more necessary to watch a speaker for visual clues. This is a good practice to continue.

6. It is not always possible to watch the speaker, for instance, on the telephone. If you practice listening to the radio when it isn't important for you to hear every word, it will give you confidence in letting your ears

work alone. Over a period of time, your telephone skills will also improve.

7. If you are not wearing two hearing instruments, you may not have your sense of direction. Although you can hear the voice clearly, you may not be able to tell exactly where the sound is coming from. It is necessary to watch the speaker to follow the flow of conversation.

USE TIME

Patience is your most important ally. **Wear your hearing instrument on a regular, daily basis. When the hearing instrument begins to make you feel tired or nervous, turn it off and remove it for a few hours. Then put it back on again.** You'll find the length of time you wear it grows, and the rest periods become fewer. Don't regress into a quiet world by going without the instrument for long periods.

In just a few weeks, you'll be able to wear it from morning until night without fatigue or nervousness. In fact, you'll really miss it when you forget to put it on.

There are a few things to check before you come back next week.

1. **Comfort.** The hearing instrument should be comfortable. No sore spots. Please call if you experience any irritation. Do not wait for a week and try to get used to sore spots. Phone and come in sooner.

2. **Echo.** Your voice should change, but it should not echo, or vibrate, or sound hollow, unless you have the hearing instrument set too loud. If you cannot get rid of the echo until sound is too quiet, come in for an adjustment.

3. **Noise.** Noise should be loud, but not uncomfortable. If you find you're reaching for the volume control because noises are too sharp, phone immediately.

BINAURAL AMPLIFICATION

Binaural hearing gives you several advantages.

1. You do not have a poor hearing side. You don't move people over to your 'good' ear. You hear from both sides.

2. You have your sense of direction. You can locate the sound source. Background noise comes from a different spot than the voice you focus on.

3. You wear two instruments quieter than only one. Clarity improves and background noise is lower.

4. You can be 'bionic' at will. For instance, as a passenger in the car, turn the right instrument, next to the traffic, off. You hear the driver better without picking up as much road and traffic noise.

5. When both ears work together, clarity and ease of listening increase.

6. People find their balance, while walking, improves. You tend to walk to the better hearing side when wearing only one instrument.

DISCRIMINATION SCORES

One of the easiest ways for the patient to associate an improvement in hearing is with speech discrimination tests. Comparison unaided or with the old hearing instrument(s), and with the new fitting vividly show the patient what differences to expect. This is your last chance to do sound field testing with the old hearing instrument. If you didn't do discrimination testing last visit, do it now. Lesson 23 discusses sound field verification.

CLIENT CARE and HEARING INSTRUMENT MAINTENANCE

Always remove your hearing instrument when:
- washing your face, hair or shaving.
- under a hair dryer.
- using hair spray or powder.
- brushing your hair.
- pulling a sweater or other garment over your head.
- showering, bathing or swimming.

Open battery door at night.

Don't put your hearing instrument near heat, in direct sunlight, or in the glove compartment of your car.

Remove wax from ITE or canal instruments only with special tool provided. Wipe the instrument with a soft cloth or tissue.

Protect your instrument from dropping or hard knocks by handling it over a table or counter, or sitting on the bed.

Use a DRI-AID kit or silica gel when moisture or perspiration is a problem.

Do not attempt to repair, lubricate or oil the hearing instrument. Take the hearing instrument in for regular service checks.

Report any change of hearing, hearing instrument function, or ability to handle the instrument.

Have regular maintenance and check-ups every four to six months.

EARMOLD

Keep the earmold free of wax. Use a wax loop. Be careful not to force the wax up the tubing. (Toothpicks are bad for this. Small pieces of wood break off and plug the tube or cause the sound to flutter).

Remove moisture bubbles or steam in the tubing whenever it occurs. Separate the earmold and tubing from the earhook. Blow through the tubing with a rubber forced air blower bulb.

When you use your mouth to blow the moisture out, your hot, moist breath turns the tube white. It returns to normal after a few seconds. Wait until the tube clears before attaching it to the hearing instrument.

Come in for a tubing change whenever

a) tubing starts to harden or deteriorate.

b) tubing separates from either hearing instrument or earmold.

c) tubing discolors, twists, splits, feels too short or too long.

d) earmold hurts, works out of ear, does not seat properly in ear, likes to feedback for any reason.

BATTERIES

Use only fresh batteries.

Store batteries in a cool, dry place, like your purse or the dresser drawer - not the fridge or freezer.

Do not leave a dead battery in the hearing instrument, or store the hearing instrument with a battery in it if you only wear the hearing instrument occasionally. It corrodes, damaging the battery contacts. Discard or recycle spent batteries.

Wipe off the battery periodically if exposed to rain, high humidity or perspiration build-up.

Do not put zinc-air batteries in DRI-AID kit. Make sure battery surface is free of glue from the tab when you insert it in the hearing instrument.

Use a battery tester after removing the hearing instrument for the night, not prior to use in the morning. Weak batteries recover some voltage overnight, but only perform for a short period after recovery. Discard a weak battery after testing. Do not save it until morning.

DO REQUIRED PAPERWORK

Fill out guarantees, warranty cards, review instruction booklet(s), etc. Discuss batteries, what the package looks like, how you get into the package, how long a battery should last, size and color code. Collect money.

Ideally, make one appointment within the first week, and another as necessary. Record these dates on a special appointment card or the back of your business card.

Verification procedures check the accuracy of your fitting. Measurements allow you to make informed adjustments or modifications, and demonstrate your patient's improvement in both hearing and understanding.

A patient who has never worn a hearing instrument benefits from a few days practical experience in handling and use before making 'fine tuning' adjustments to the fitting. Some previous users require practice time, too, while others relish anything you want to do or measure. For them, the verification is part of the fitting process, and may be the reason for the new hearing instrument(s).

For those who require time, your patient interview checks their progress. The reactions and experiences guide you in further adjustments or modifications.

Write down every complaint and every advantage. The complaints usually demonstrate a specific problem, described several ways. For instance, if a larger vent is required, they won't like something about their voice, background noise or car noise will be on the list, they will talk about echo and vibration, the ear feels full and other people's voices sound harsh. The patient cannot stand the sound when they chew.

VERIFICATION

When you verify a fitting, you reinforce the patient's improvement in various conditions in a tangible, measureable way. Results support the patient's decision to use amplification, encourage both the patient and family members to become involved again, enhance communication, and return confidence and self-esteem. The fact that the verification is measurable, not just something the patient perceives, cements the decision to wear hearing instruments.

Hearing instruments do not cure hearing loss, or return thresholds to normal range, or make you hear and understand normally. Hearing instruments do help hearing loss, improve thresholds, and help you to communicate easier.

Normal range is 0 - 20 dB HL. Thresholds are not in normal range, but thresholds do improve. Verification shows us how much we improve the threshold, not whether we return the range to normal. If we return the lower frequencies to normal, the upward spread of masking affects the higher frequencies. We purposefully bleed off lower frequencies by venting, and tilt the frequency response to accent the highs. We sometimes do improve thresholds to the outer limits of normal range, but this is not our ultimate goal in the fitting.

If we have not taken aided thresholds into our definition of normal range, then the aided PTA and aided SRT cannot possibly be in normal range either. But, because impaired hearing thresholds have abnormal loudness growth, we hope to prove MCL is comfortable for the patient and understandable at normal presentation levels. UCL does not change whether the patient is aided or unaided. Our verification measurements prove we have not exceeded UCL.

SOUND FIELD AUDIOMETRY

Any area with sound waves present is a sound field, where sound reflects and bounces freely. A 'live' room is highly reverberant. Free field is a large outdoor area with no surfaces to reflect sound. An anechoic chamber approximates a free field, without reflections or echoes. A free field or 'dead' room requires special treatment to stop reverberation.

FUNCTIONAL GAIN

When adding amplification to a patient with a hearing loss, we expect each of our unaided test results to change.

We can predict, or calculate a change, using PMI test results or functional gain requirements. Based on our predicted or calculated change, we select and fit a hearing instrument/earmold combination. Sound field testing measures the change to prove the hearing instrument and earmold fitting are as good as, or better than, our predictions or calculations.

AIDED and UNAIDED AUDIOMETRIC THRESHOLDS

Verify your aided threshold prediction by sound field audiometry. You require external speakers, either calibrated to the audiometer, or with correction factors to add or subtract at each frequency. Follow the manufacturer's instructions for speaker distance and angle, in a sound field.

Depending on the loss, you may need to either plug the non-test ear, or use masking without occluding the test ear.

SPEECH AUDIOMETRY

Because sound field speech measurements approximate 'real life' situations, they should be in a sound field rather than a controlled environment like a sound booth. Speaker placement for speech audiometry should be 0° and one (1) meter.

Speech tests measured through the audiometer circuit determine the levels in HL. Speech tests at the same intensity, using a sound level meter at the microphone of the hearing instrument in SPL are 20 dB higher. Remember, ANSI Standards add 20 dB to convert speech from HL to SPL. You must subtract 20 dB if you use the audiometer circuit in sound field.

Measure the discrimination words in sound field at the microphone of the hearing instrument if you use a tape recorder and speaker separate from the audiometer. The measurements, in SPL, remain constant for unaided, old instrument and new instrument tests.

AIDED SPEECH RECEPTION THRESHOLD

A relationship exists between poor discrimination scores and the impaired unaided or aided speech reception threshold. Poor scores penalize the hearing instrument performance, but there is a difference between SAT and SRT. SRT requires hearing and understanding. Regardless of what you want to measure, MCL is where the patient consistently turns the volume of the hearing instrument.

AIDED SPEECH DISCRIMINATION SCORES

This simulates normal conversational position in a real life situation. Use a recorded presentation level of 50 - 70 dBA, measured at the microphone of the hearing instrument in SPL. 50 dB SPL represents a very quiet conversational level. Audiometer presentation levels are 30 -50 dB HL.

With the hearing instrument turned to the patient's comfortable level, present 25 recorded NU 6 or other Discrimination words in sound field at your predetermined level. Binaural discrimination scores should be as good or better than the better ear score.

SIGNAL TO NOISE (S/N) RATIO

Patients prefer recorded Discrimination Tests at 10 dB S/N for average environment. A 10 dB S/N means the words are 10 dB louder than the background noise. Most children under ten years old, and normal adults over fifty, require a signal to noise advantage for good discrimination scores.

UCL'S

Exposure to high levels of sound with the instrument at a use setting provides proof the fitting gives adequate protection, without exceeding the patient's tolerance or speech interference levels.

COMFORT

Comfort does not mean fit, alone. It can mean a lack of dexterity with the controls, or sensitivity in the fingertips. Noise creates discomfort, anxiety, frustration, and emotional outbreaks. Discomfort includes hearing yourself chew too loud, your voice sounding hoarse or tinny or vibrating when you talk. When you feel like you're coming down with a cold while you wear the hearing instrument, comfort is the relief you have when you take it off. Feedback is uncomfortable, quietness, blessed.

PROBE MICROPHONE VERIFICATION

We worked with 'functional gain' and 'use gain' as it relates to unaided and aided threshold measurements. When we use an instrument with a probe microphone tip in the ear canal, functional gain and use gain become **insertion gain.**

The measurements cover two categories - a gain change in the ear canal, or a response change of the hearing instrument because of resonances and vents.

EAR CANAL RESONANCE

REUR: Real ear unaided response - the measured frequency response in dB SPL with a probe tube microphone in the unaided, unoccluded ear canal.

INSERTION LOSS

REOR: Real Ear Occluded Response measures the frequency response in dB SPL with a probe microphone in the ear canal, with the earmold in place, and the hearing instrument turned 'off'. This measurement demonstrates direct acoustic input to the ear canal through a vent or slit leak. It also demonstrates resonances created by an interaction between the earmold vent and residual effective canal volume.

INSERTION RESPONSE

REIR: Real Ear Insertion Response is the mathematical difference between the REAR and REUR when both are measured at the same point in the canal with the same sound field. i.e., REAR - REUR = REIR. REIR is insertion gain in dB comparing the aided condition to the unaided condition without including the input.

AIDED RESPONSE

REAR: Real Ear Aided Response represents the in situ aided frequency response measured in dB SPL with a probe tube microphone in the aided external auditory canal.

In situ describes the hearing instrument response, while other measurements describe the changes in the ear canal.

REIG: Real Ear Insertion Gain is the REAR - REUR differences measured at a specified frequency. REIR and REIG are relative measures with zero (0) indicating no difference between the unaided and aided sound pressure levels.

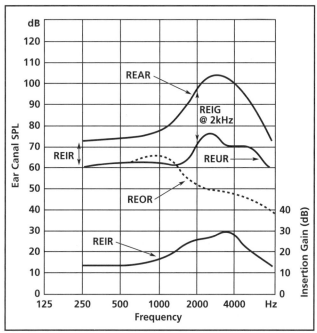

Fig. 26-1
Probe Measurement Responses

Real ear measurements do not replace patient feedback. Just because things look good at the eardrum, it doesn't mean the processing at the brain is ideal, or that middle ear function is what you expect. Do not get so involved in your prescription, or your computor screen that you forget who you intend to help.

INTERNATIONAL INSTITUTE FOR HEARING INSTRUMENTS STUDIES

DISTANCE LEARNING for Professionals in HEARING HEALTH SCIENCES

REAL EAR MEASUREMENT

LESSON 28

In Lesson 26 you learned fitting verification can be accomplished by several different methods. This verification process is critically important as technology continues to advance. Multiple Memory, Digitally Programmable, Algorithms, Analog to Digital Converters, Advanced Compression are all terms used to describe a whole new generation of hearing instruments. Without a way to accurately and repeatedly measure in-situ much of the performance these systems offer are left unrealized.

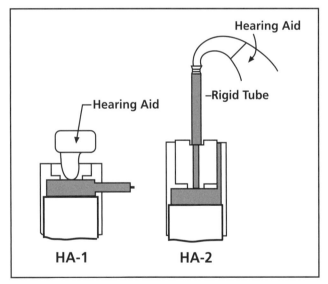

Fig. 27-1 ANSI specified 2cc hard wall hearing aid couplers for electroacoustic measurement of hearing aid output

COUPLER HISTORY

The ANSI S3.22 standard mandates that hearing aid performance be made in a 2-cm3 coupler. Romanow developed this test method in 1942 as a temporary way for manufacturers to verify the response of a particular model hearing aid. This coupler has no correlation to the real human ear and was never intended to simulate

it, but only designed as a quality control tool for hearing aid manufacturers. Romanow suggested that correction factors could be applied to the 2-cm3 coupler to more closely resemble the ear. It's ironic that a temporary test method developed over 50 years ago is still the standard the industry uses today.

Zwislocki in 1970, '71 proposed a physical cavity that more closely resembles the human ear. This method however does not take into consideration the diffraction of sound caused by head shadow, the Pinna or ear canal characteristics.

A realistic manikin known as Knowles Electronic Manikin for Acoustic Research (KEMAR) was a major development in the mid 1970's. KEMAR allowed hearing aid manufacturers to reliably and repeatedly test hearing aid performance in a near real world environment. KEMAR is still used extensively in the development and testing of hearing aid performance. However, it is based on median anthropomorphic values from adults and does not provide specific data for an individual, which can deviate substantially from KEMAR.

It has always been the goal to measure hearing instrument response close to the Tympanic Membrane (TM). As early as 1946 Weiner and Ross used fixed probe measurements to evaluate real ear responses. Clinical application of Probe-Microphone measurements did not take place until the late 1970's when Hartford and Preves proposed what today is the modern REAL EAR MEASUREMENT system. Rastronics released the first commercial unit in December of 1983, (the CCI-10).

SYSTEM FUNCTION

All Real Ear Measurement (REM) systems have the same basic pieces. That is not to say they are all created alike. Every system is based upon a computer processor, some are dedicated to only one function, others are pieces of hardware and programs that are added to an existing computer. Just like different computer programs, the controls and operations vary by manufacturer. All REM's have a signal generator that produces sounds. These can be unique product noise bursts or clicks; the industry has standardized several different types of signals. These sounds or noises are equalized by a reference microphone, which makes sure the sound being analyzed by the computer stays at the correct intensity. A measurement microphone is attached to a soft silicone probe tube, which is inserted into the ear canal near the TM. The acoustic signals picked up by the probe tube microphone are analyzed by a computer and displayed as curves. These curves, known as responses, are sent to some type of display device.

SIGNAL TYPES

Early systems only used a Swept tone, either pure or warble, for measurements. Later generations added numerous other types of noises including clicks, narrowband noise bursts, wide band noise, and several different types of speech noise weighted signals. Most modern systems offer a choice in the type of signal available. There is a clear advantage to using some type of speech weighted noise, especially for compression instruments.

SPEAKER PLACEMENT

The signal is directed to a speaker, which can be placed at different angles to the ear under test. Studies by Killion and Revit indicate a speaker azimuth of 45° to be the most reliable for test re-test variability. A 0° placement

is usually more practical in the normal test environment. (Whichever placement is chosen, the specialist needs to be aware that different Sound Pressure Levels (SPL) will be recorded as the speaker placement changes. It is important to use the same speaker position or set up for all measurements.)

PROBE MICROPHONE HOUSING

The signals are measured by a reference microphone, which is usually, but not always, attached to the Probe Tube coupler housing. The job of the reference microphone is to make sure any changes in room noise or head movement allows the system to update the signal being delivered to the speaker.

Attached to the measurement microphone is a soft silicone Probe Tube, which is inserted into the ear canal and picks up the sound near the TM.

PROBE TUBE PLACEMENT

The most critical measurement variable in REM is probe tube placement. As the probe tube is moved in relationship to the TM, Standing Waves located along the ear canal can change the measured SPL verses actual TM SPL by as much as 12dB (and in some rare cases even more). As illustrated in fig. 27-3, a distance of 10mm from the TM can create a standing wave error of 10dB SPL at 8,000 Hz and 5dB at 6,000 Hz. When a distance of 5mm from the TM is achieved, the accuracy of the measurement is within 2dB through 8,000 Hz.

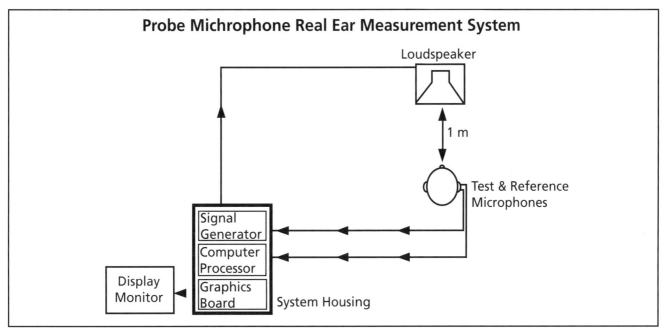

Fig. 27-2 Block diagram of typical Probe Microphone Real Ear Measurement System

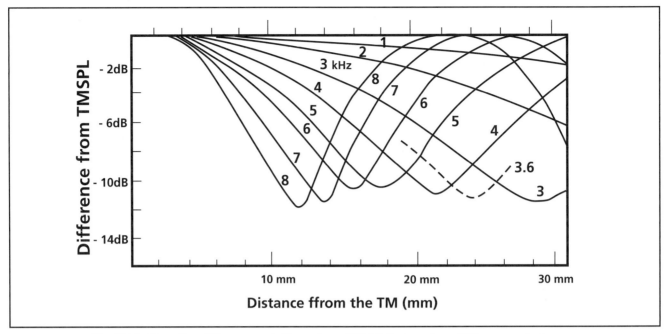

Fig. 27-3 Standing Wave graph (based on KEMAR) showing differences between TM SPL and Probe Tube SPL as a function of distance and frequency

It is also important that the probe tube tip is well past the end of the ear mold. As illustrated in Fig. 27-4. at a distance of less than 5mm from the end of the ear mold, large discrepancies can occur.

Positioning the Probe Tube takes practice. The easiest way is to view the canal with an Otoscope taking note of the ear canal depth. Mark the Probe Tube at 30mm (most tubes have a ring that slides) from the end of the tip, insert the probe tip into the canal with a slight twisting motion and locate the mark at the Intertragal notch. This should place the tip between 5 to 15mm from the TM. Perform a Real Ear Unaided Response (REUR) and observe the result on the display. If a response at 6,000

Hz occurs below the input level, advance the tube by 3mm. If the response at 6,000 Hz. increases above the input level, remark the probe tube and perform the rest of the tests. If not, continue to gently advance the probe tube until the response at 6,000 Hz is above the input level. Stop advancing the probe tube if the test subject reports hearing a thud or complains of discomfort.

It is important to note that the insertion of the probe tube will not damage a normal TM if tip comes in contact with it, however, some individuals report discomfort upon insertion of the probe tube. Consideration of the test subjects comfort should always take precedence over ideal probe tube location.

DISPLAY

The computer's processor then analyzes the results. These results are saved or recorded as different responses depending on the type of measurement being performed. Usually the responses, which resemble 2cc coupler curves, are displayed on a monitor in line graph form with frequency on the X-axis and intensity on the Y-axis. Some of the displays are multi-color large screens; others can be small monochrome displays. Most REM's allow hard copies to be generated. Some even will save results to a client specific database for future recall.

Notes should be kept on every measurement for speaker azimuths, signal used, probe tube depth, and test environments for recall at a later date if measurements are to be repeated.

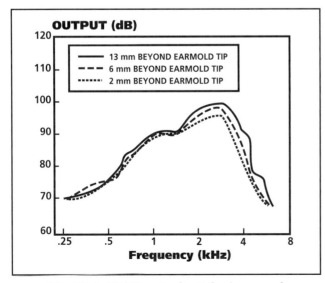

Fig. 27-4 REAR as Probe Tube is moved in relationship to end of ear mold

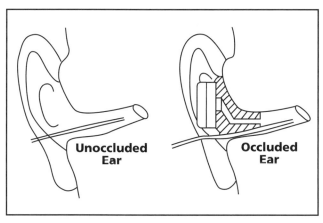

Fig. 27-5 Proper Probe Tube placement in the ear

TEST ENVIRONMENTS

A Sound Booth is the preferred location for REM, however, that is not always available. A sound treated suite can be a good alternative. REM can even be performed in a quiet living room. Whichever location is used the following considerations should always be followed.

The loudspeaker is positioned about one meter from the test subject. The ambient noise level in the room should not be excessive compared to the signal level (most systems require the noise floor to be 10dB less than the measured signal). No reflective surfaces should be within 2 meters of the ear being measured.

SIGNAL LEVELS

Most REM's are capable of signals between 50 and 90dB SPL. The level used will vary depending on the test. REUR's should be between 60 to 70dB SPL while Real Ear Saturation Responses (RESR) can be as high as 90dB SPL. Many hearing instruments with compression circuits need to be measured both before and after compression takes place. Keeping in mind that several popular hearing instrument circuits start compression at 45dB SPL but is rarely possible to measure a level below 55dB SPL due to the noise floor in most test environments. Preferably a family of curves for Real Ear Aided Responses (REAR) should be run, especially for newer advanced compression instruments, so changes in performance can be observed.

SIGNAL TIME

The first several generations of REM's available only offered a swept tone measurement of some type. This means that a hearing instrument with any type of frequency dependent compression would be in compression for part of the sweep and out of compression for the remainder. A system that delivers real time (all frequencies measured at the same instant) is essential for anything other than straight linear instruments. This is often referred to as Fast Fourier Transform (FFT). REM's that use FFT can show all three dimensions of acoustics; frequency, amplitude and time, all at once on a single display.

PRESCRIPTIVE METHODS

Much is written on different prescription formulas, with arguments both for and against. It is important to remember that a perfect target match is rarely obtainable for any formula. Even if obtained, the test subject may still not be able to tolerate the end result. A target is something you try to approximate and a good place to start the fitting process.

Prescriptive methods are divided into two categories, Linear and Non-Linear. There are times when it would be desirable to use one method and prescription over another. As illustrated in Fig. 27-7 large differences do occur in formula targets. The more severe the loss the more aggressive should be the target. Keep in mind, a sensorineural loss does not need as much gain as a conductive loss. Generally it is up to the specialist to choose one of their liking.

LINEAR FORMULAS

Linear formulas such as NAL, Berger, POGO, Libby, 1/2 Gain, 1/3 Gain, etc. all prescribe different levels of amplification for different frequencies. No one formula has been documented to be universally superior to the other. Linear formulas should ONLY be applied to linear instruments.

NON-LINEAR FORMULAS

Non-Linear formulas such as DSL(I/O), Fig. 27-6, Pasco, and IHAFF access performance by frequency and intensity. The vast majority of the hearing impaired population does not need as much amplification for a loud sound as they do for a soft one. It is not necessary to target the same amount of gain for 85 to 90dB SPL, as it is for 50 to 60dB SPL. Several non-linear formulas use published norms as their targets for different inputs, some are designed specifically for Wide Band compression circuits while others are formulated for higher compression thresholds. DSL(I/O) is designed primarily for children while IHAFF takes into consideration individual Loudness Growth with a method for the test subject to choose levels they prefer.

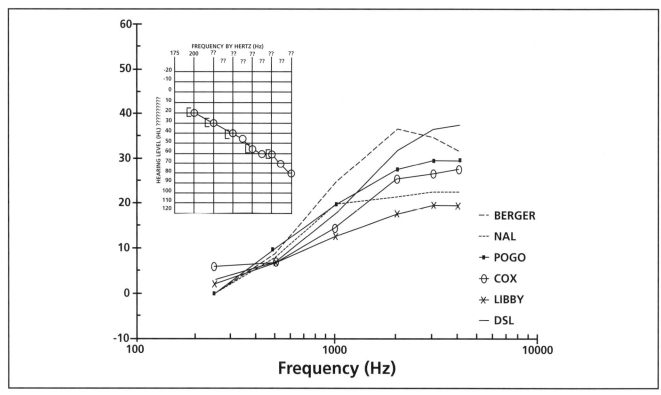

Fig. 27-6 Prescribed REIR targets for six different formulas using the same hearing loss

Always listen to what the individual tells you! The reason REM is so important is that the response of a hearing instrument in the ear is unique to the individual. The industry is geared to fitting the individual, their needs and desires can never be replaced by scientific calculations or published norms. REM provides an objective, repeatable measurement of hearing instrument performance. It allows the specialist to view fitting problems and the effects of any changes made.

TEST BATTERIES
REUR *Real Ear Unaided Response*

The REUR is a measurement of SPL, as a function of frequency, at a specified point in the unoccluded ear canal for a specified soundfield. This can be expressed in SPL or as gain in decibels relative to the stimulus level.

The REUR is used as a reference value for the calculation of insertion gain. All REUR's are unique to the individual even though many REUR's resemble that of KEMAR; most show differences, some large and some very small. The REUR is the individual's natural amplification which they have had most of their life. Additionally, there is a direct decibel for decibel relationship between Real Ear Insertion Response (REIR) and REUR.

TEST PROTOCOL

1. Place the probe tube into the ear canal to a proper insertion depth as described previously.

2. Choose the stimulus type (preferably some type of speech weighted noise) and intensity (60 to 70dB SPL). Be sure to use the same stimulus type for all measurements.

3. Conduct measurement.

REOR *Real Ear Occluded Response*

The REOR is a measurement of SPL, as a function of frequency, at a specified point in the ear canal for a specified soundfield, with the hearing aid in place and turned off. This can be expressed in SPL or as gain in decibels relative to the stimulus level.

The effect of placing a hearing instrument in a patient's ear alters the natural open ear response, creating an insertion loss. The tighter the fit, smaller the vent, or longer the canal, the greater the insertion loss and lower the REOR will be on the SPL chart. The REOR is useful in measuring the Helmholtz Resonance of the vent and verifying the tightness of the ear mold fitting.

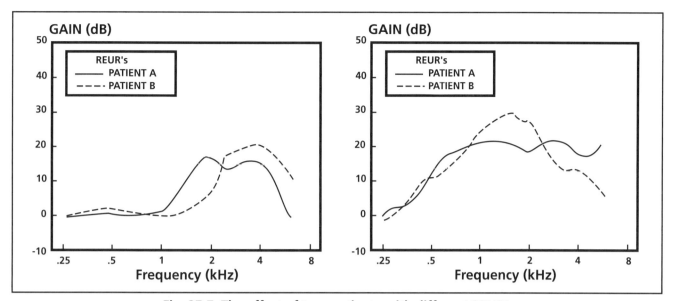

Fig. 27-7 The effect of two patients with different REUR's on the REIR measured with the same instrument

TEST PROTOCOL

1. Place the probe tube into the ear canal as it was for the REUR.

2. Choose the stimulus type. Be sure to use the same stimulus type used in the REUR.

3. Insert the instrument into the ear canal with power turned off.

4. Conduct measurement.

REAR *Real Ear Aided Response*

The REAR is a measurement of SPL, as a function of frequency, at a specified point in the ear canal for a specified soundfield, with the hearing aid in place and turned on. This can be expressed in SPL or as gain in decibels relative to the stimulus level.

The REAR uses the individual's ear canal as the coupler and all the effects of the fitting can be seen including the venting, tightness of fit, and appropriateness of the amplification. REAR is especially useful in trouble shooting user complaints by observing the response in different frequency bands where the individual may be experiencing problems. (E.g. Complaints of tinniness may be due to spikes in the high frequencies, or excessive background noise due to too much low frequency amplification.)

The REAR is also used in determining the REIR, with the REAR the upper level and REUR the lower. (REIR=REAR-REUR). With the advent of modern advanced compression, more emphasis is being placed on the importance of REAR. Families of REAR curves are used to determine the effects of intensity increases on compression circuitry fittings, which can be an important fitting tool.

TEST PROTOCOL

1. Place the probe tube into the ear canal as it was for the REUR.

2. Choose the stimulus type. Be sure to use the same stimulus type used in the REUR.

3. Insert the instrument into the ear canal with power turned on to the desired volume control position.

4. Conduct measurements at a single level using the same level and stimulus used for the REUR. A variety of levels starting at 50 to 60dB SPL and increasing in 5 to 10dB steps ending at 85 or 90dB SPL, can be used to observe the Knee Point and Compression Ratios in advanced fittings.

RESR *Real Ear Saturation Response*

The RESR is a measurement of SPL, as a function of frequency, at a specified point in the ear canal for a specified soundfield, with the hearing aid in place and turned on. This response differs from the REAR in that the measurement is obtained with the stimulus level sufficiently intense as to operate the hearing aid at its maximum output level approximately 85 to 90dB SPL.

The RESR is the total output a hearing aid is capable of producing in the ear, similar to the ANSI SSPL-90 coupler measurement. It is a desirable measurement for linear fittings, but has been replaced by a family of REAR curves for compression instruments. Verifying a fitting that is both safe and one that will not exceed the individuals level of discomfort is one of the primary goals in all fittings.

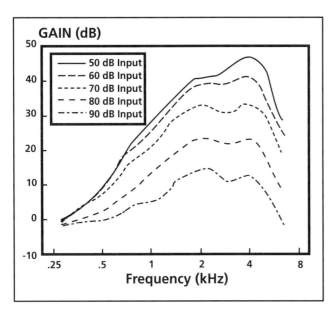

Fig. 27-8 Family of REIR curves as input is increased from 50 to 90dB for a compression circuit

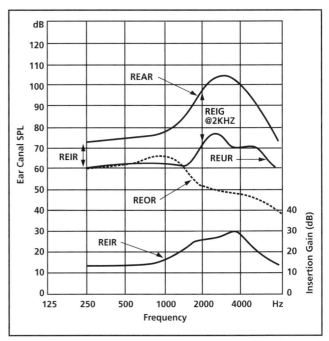

Fig. 27-9 Real Ear Response Curves

TEST PROTOCOL

1. Place the probe tube into the ear canal to a proper depth.

2. Choose the stimulus type.

3. Insert the instrument into the ear canal with power turned on to a level just below feedback.

4. Conduct measurement at 85 to 90dB or enough to saturate the instrument.

REIR *Real Ear Insertion Response*

The REIR is the difference in decibels as a function of frequency, between the REUR and REAR measurements, taken at the same point in the same soundfield.

The REIR is the amount of gain delivered at the TM. It is also referred to as functional gain and is similar to the frequency response measurement as specified by ANSI. Its primary purpose is to compare actual measurements to a desired target. At one time it was the most used measurement in assessment of linear instrument fittings. Currently, with the advent of advanced compression fittings, its importance is questionable.

TEST PROTOCOL

1. Place the probe tube into the ear canal as it was for the REUR.

2. Choose the stimulus type. Be sure to use the same stimulus type used in REUR.

3. Insert the instrument into the ear canal with volume control adjusted to the desired level.

4. Conduct measurement.

The REIG Real Ear Insertion Gain is the value, in decibels, of the REIR at a specific frequency. (E.g. 25dB of Real Ear Insertion Gain at 3500 Hz.) Fig. 27-9 illustrates a response graph with the entire family of Real ear curves displayed.

POST FITTING CARE; FOLLOW-UP AND REHABILITATION

LESSON 29

Post fitting care is often the single most significant factor in hearing instrument acceptance and use. Patient instruction, assessing patient responses, counselling, rehabilitation concepts, and family member interaction are necessary ongoing processes.

Aural rehabilitation, another name for follow up care, automatically becomes part of every visit, - questions, education, communication tips, and encouragement all help the patient to accept hearing instruments as a positive experience.

Help the patient understand the physical loss. Deal with the psychological and social reaction to hearing loss. This is a giant step toward accepting methods of coping with the patient's impairment. Keep the patient's expectations within realistic bounds.

As the patient goes through the adaptation process, many questions, problems, and fitting procedures require more knowledge on the patient's part. This guiding process always expands limits, attitudes, and motivation.

Encourage family involvement, beginning with the initial testing, and continuing with the follow-up sessions and regular check-ups. Hearing loss definitely effects their behavior, attitudes and interactions. You avoid unreasonable expectations or misconceptions when they, too, become involved in the patient's rehabilitation. Keep them informed too, using pamphlets, letters, cards, etc. with short tips or instructions aimed at them.

Friends and family want to talk with hard of hearing people, but they do not know how. They assume hearing loss means loss of volume, rather than discrimination, so they talk loudly.

On the other hand, many hearing impaired people do not know what helps them to hear better, so they fail to make suggestions. Communication truly is a two-way street. It requires effort from both parties.

Improve communication with special speaking skills. Hearing impaired people need to combine visual clues to increase what they do hear. Encourage family and friends to meet this specific need.

HOW to HAVE SUCCESSFUL FOLLOW-UP CARE

Schedule periodic hearing instrument performance checks. Encourage the patient to contact you when any change in hearing levels is noticed, for whatever reason. The patient may adapt to negative changes without knowing it, and regress to a far less effective hearing instrument use. They only compare the way they hear today with the response yesterday, or last week.

Some changes occur slowly, over time. The patient may blame their hearing loss, not the hardened tube, or corroded battery contacts, etc. Send service reminders every four to six months. You expect your dentist or optometrist to remind you to have check-ups. You are as important to your patient.

The physical condition and the condition of the patient's ear undergo changes too, like irritation, impacted wax, changes in health, dental health, weight, and medications. Each affect their hearing, their hearing instrument, and their communication skills. These changes require retesting, adjustments and modifications. Your questions and discussions at each check-up guide you.

An 'ideal' approach to post fitting care involves other professionals who can benefit the patient – doctors, psychologists, social workers, vocational counselors, audiologists, hard of hearing self-help groups, tinnitus associations, or others relating to the particular loss and medical problem.

HEARING ENHANCEMENT TIPS
with or without the HEARING INSTRUMENT

Often the problem the patient experiences relates to room acoustics more than hearing loss. When the patient is wearing their hearing instrument in public, the acoustic characteristics vary greatly.

Explain the following to your client:

1. Sound travels in all directions and bounces off whatever surface it hits. A large room, or a room with a high ceiling, creates a difficult listening area in the center of the room. They hear better nearer a wall.

2. An archway or doorway transforms two smaller rooms into one large room. The patient should move a few feet away from the opening and avoid these acoustic effects.

3. Sound bounces off shiny surfaces like mirrors and windows, and is absorbed by soft or dull surfaces. It is easier to hear when sound is absorbed. Closing the drapes makes a big difference when sitting in front of a window. The patient hears better in a living room with rugs, drapes, soft furniture, etc., than in the kitchen with enamel surfaces, shiny walls and tile floors.

4. They also hear better in a high backed chair than a low one - like cupping the hand behind the ear, the sound stops at the chair back.

5. The patient should experiment at church, concerts, the theater, by sitting in different places. Find out which seating location has the best acoustics. For instance, when the Minister stands at a raised pulpit, the voice carries right over their head when sitting too close. When lipreading skills are more important, sitting closer provides a better view of the speaker.

6. The patient should avoid sitting next to a wall or ceiling mounted speaker. Vibration from the speaker distorts the sound.

MAINTENANCE, MODIFICATIONS AND REPAIR

LESSON 30

Once the patient becomes a hearing instrument user, the importance of proper maintenance and operation are critical factors in their daily communication. The patient may have lived without the hearing instrument for many years, but now any time without their hearing instrument may cause great discomfort.

Be thorough in your instructions to the patient during the fitting process. Remind them of things they can do when they come in for their check ups. Diligently do your maintenance tasks. Ask health related questions each time you see the patient. Record volume control settings so you know when their requirements change.

If you detect and head off problems, make adjustments as thresholds change, correct minor repairs yourself, spot factory repair situations, and supply them with a loaner hearing instrument while their instrument is sent to the manufacturer for repair, the patients need to be secure in their ability to hear and communicate will be fulfilled.

DISPENSER MAINTENANCE BATTERIES

Always use a fresh battery for maintenance checks, or test the patient's battery under load to see if it maintains current and voltage levels.

A weak battery gives all sorts of misleading results. Patient complaints include:

1. Not enough gain.
2. Output lower than normal.
3. Distortion, scratchy, hollow sound, muffled, echo, poor sound quality.
4. Buzzing, motorboating, oscillation, dead.
5. Intermittent, noisy.
6. Works, then dies. Works again several hours later, but dies quickly.

BATTERY CONTACTS

Clean battery contacts with a pencil eraser or the flat side of a wooden toothpick. To check battery contacts, if the hearing instrument has a telecoil, switch the telephone coil on and volume control at low. If you hear a click, the controls are OK. Raise battery contacts if they do not apply a slight pressure to the battery. (Many dead hearing instruments only require lifting the battery contacts).

Check the battery door. The battery fits in easily and the door opens and closes without binding, but does not fall open on its own. Battery brands differ slightly in height. If the battery seems higher or lower than the case, try a different brand.

MICROPHONE and RECEIVER

Check both the microphone and receiver openings for wax, skin oils, moisture, perspiration, ear discharge, etc. Hold the sound bore upside down while cleaning so debris falls out of the opening.

When you clean the receiver tubing (out of sight of the patient), modify a wax loop. Cut one side of the loop free. Straighten it out. Then form a small hook on the tip. Look down the sound bore with an otoscope. The receiver looks black, and any wax shows up well in the light. Wax, draining ears, and ear drops or salve may plug receivers. Hairspray, cosmetics, and perspiration can clog microphones.

To check the receiver and microphone, turn the hearing instrument on to the telephone coil, with volume low. The receiver is okay if you hear amplification. Switch to the (M) microphone position. If you do not hear your voice amplify, the problem is the microphone.

Also reference the section in this lesson on Feedback regarding binding microphones and receivers, and the use of windscreens.

VOLUME CONTROL

Each side of the volume control accumulates dirt and perspiration. Debris builds up near user level because the volume control setting stays relatively the same from day to day. The dirt causes a dead spot or static both above and below the use setting when turning the volume up or down. Rotate the volume control several times to wear down or lift out the dirty area.

If this is not sufficient, use a small drop of electronic contact cleaner. DO NOT spray cleaner into the volume control. Check the complete volume control rotation while listening for static, dead spots or distortion. Wiggle the control from side to side, and push it in gently as you're turning. Feedback cuts in and out during these motions with a faulty volume control. The volume control and off/on switch fail through constant use.

Sometimes, the control separates from the faceplate. The entire control rotates. Each turn of the control twists the wires inside the case. When this occurs, send the hearing instrument to the manufacturer for repair.

When patients have difficulty finding or adjusting the volume control on in-the-ear (ITE) or canal instruments, stack the volume control with another cap. The double cap sticks out far enough that they can locate it; and they can turn the wheel easily using both their thumb and finger. This may assist those patients with a lack of sensitivity in the fingertips.

AMPLIFIER

The amplifier is working properly when you hear terminal noise with the volume control on low. The first amplifier is functioning properly when noise varies on the telecoil.

SWITCHES

Check **switches** in each position. Wiggle the switch as you change positions, but do not force it past the setting. The switch is faulty if you hear circuit or background noise in the off position. Off is silent, with no sound at all.

The **telephone coil** buzzes, and the buzz increases with volume control rotation. (It also buzzes near fluorescent lights or appliances like an electric kettle). A faulty telephone coil sounds like a functioning off-switch.

A **noise suppressor switch** is easiest to check in noise, but also changes the quality of your voice. Without changing the volume wheel, the volume decreases when the switch is in active suppression because the low frequencies reduce.

ADJUSTMENT POTENTIOMETERS

Malfunctioning **adjustment potentiomenters (pots)** show little or no change over the range of the control, or, at some settings the instrument sounds weak or dead. Listen to the feedback of the hearing instrument as you rotate throughout the range of the potentiometer. Move the faulty control back and forth several times, or use a drop of alcohol or electronic cleaner to clean the pot. If this does not correct the problem, send the hearing instrument to the manufacturer for repair.

WIRING

To detect wiring problems, turn the hearing instrument full-on. Twist, tap, and squeeze the case. A short circuit, loose wire, or poor solder connection shows up as intermittent feedback. The weakest link is the microphone wiring.

When **instrument works with battery door slightly open,** but stops when door is closed properly, receiver posts need further insulation, or loose wires behind the battery area touch the battery and short out when the door closes. You can easily see these wires. Move them out of the way.

EAR HOOK or COUPLER

Put instrument on telecoil and the volume at low. If you hear a click, the ear hook is working properly. Replace the plugged hook when you do not hear a click.

MEASUREMENTS and LISTENING TESTS

Run a listening check on the hearing instrument. Graph the acoustic output of the hearing instrument with a hearing instrument analyzer at either the user level or ANSI Standards for hearing instruments. ANSI Standards tell you the instrument is within specifications. The graph from the hearing instrument analyzer will indicate if a change in the acoustic output occurs.

TEST YOUR SKILLS

Hearing instruments can have several problems, like wax in the receiver tubing, dead spots on the volume control, corrosion on battery contacts, etc. and STILL FUNCTION. Correct each item.

When you test a dead hearing instrument, more than one problem can also exist, but only one problem caused the hearing instrument to quit working.

EARMOLD

Remove the old earmold tubing, place the earmold in a ultrasonic cleaner with warm water and benzylkonium chloride. Retube the earmold using the same criteria as the original tubing, i.e., same size, ID, OD, length in sound bore, filters or dampers if any, vent drilled out (diagonal venting into sound bore). Put the hearing instrument on the patient's ear and the earmold in the ear. Cut the earmold tubing to the proper length.

ACOUSTIC MODIFICATIONS

Acoustic modifications change the frequency response of the hearing instrument. Review venting, damping, and horn effects in the lessons on hearing instruments, earmolds, and verification of hearing instrument fittings. Both venting and horn effects improve high frequency emphasis, while damping reduces peaks without having an effect on high frequency amplification.

TROUBLESHOOTING ACOUSTIC PROBLEMS

Feedback: Feedback occurs at any stage of the **fitting or follow up.** Isolating causes differ, depending on when the feedback starts. For instance, when you fit a **new hearing instrument** for the first time, you test and check the hearing instrument both with ANSI Standards for hearing instruments and listening tests. If feedback occurs at this point with an in-the-ear (ITE) or in-the-canal (ITC) instrument, one cause can be a shifted microphone or receiver.

A second cause is when the **microphone opening is too close to the volume control, tragus, or helix.** It is readily solved by adding a windscreen, or half of a windscreen, to protect the microphone from interference. Also, a small piece of foam in the microphone tubing helps. These trade-offs slightly restrict the sensitivity of the microphone. The manufacturer may need to reposition the microphone.

The **frequency response of the microphone or receiver** may cause feedback on a particular patient. Ask the hearing instrument manufacturer to advise you about a different circuit when you cannot determine the cause.

A third cause is when the **angle of the vent** allows the sound to escape, travel along the helix rim, and re-enter the microphone (with or without a windbaffle or windscreen). Remove the windbaffle. Remount it with the open end up.

High frequency peaks create feedback. Filters or dampers smooth the peaks, reducing feedback. Feedback reduction circuits or high frequency potentiometers as options on ITE or canal hearing instruments **cut the high frequencies,** reducing feedback. Resonant peak adjustment potentiometers **move the peak slightly up or down** to match ear canal resonance more accurately. Feedback reduction occurs. Gain trimmers **reduce gain across frequencies.**

High gain levels require good acoustic coupling in earmolds. Look for **earmold related problems,** first. Check fit, canal angle, mandibular motion, length of canal, venting requirements. When you are in doubt about the fit, use a temporary build up material. If this solves the problem, either build up or remake the earmold or hearing instrument.

Patients with extremely high gain hearing instruments and tight earmolds sometimes require the earmold **tubing extended to the tip of the earmold** instead of belled or flared. This reduces the gain at and above 3000 Hz, also reducing feedback. Remember to use heavy wall tubing in the earmold for this type of loss. If you replace standard wall tubing with heavy wall, ream out the sound bore to fit the outside diameter of the earmold tubing.

The solutions differ when feedback occurs **long after the patient wears hearing instruments.** First, determine if the feedback is an internal problem with the hearing instrument, or external (the coupling system), or the ear, itself.

ISOLATION of FEEDBACK PROBLEMS

A behind-the-ear (BTE) hearing instrument and attached earmold whistles with the switch on the microphone position (M) and the volume control setting at full on. Cover the tip of the earmold canal (and any diagonal vent at the external surface). The feedback should stop.

Problem is:

a. proper seating of the earmold.

b. proper fit of the earmold.

c. excess or impacted earwax.

d. change of hearing, an ear infection, or a foreign body.

e. extremely weak battery.

If feedback continues, remove the earmold and tubing from the coupler. Cover the coupler tip with your finger. Feedback should stop. The problem is earmold or earmold tubing related.

If feedback continues, remove the earhook (it usually unscrews, but some snap off). Cover receiver nubbin. DO NOT COVER MICROPHONE. When feedback stops, the earhook is split. Replace the hook. The hearing instrument has internal feedback if feedback continues. Supply the patient with a loaner hearing instrument and send the hearing instrument to the manufacturer for repair.

An ITE or canal hearing instrument has internal feedback when the receiver tubing is not entirely sealed in the sound bore, or tubing has a hole in it. Twisting and gouging with the wax loop (pick) breaks the tubing away.

Vicious cleaning methods also push the receiver tubing inside the hearing instrument. You can see the tubing, but the sound bore is empty. Give the patient another lesson in the cleaning of the hearing instrument. You can sometimes recover the tube with a modified wax loop. Patients also push the microphone into the case, thinking they need to clean the opening. This usually requires returning the hearing instrument to the manufacturer for repair.

Another cause of internal feedback is a hole from the vent into the case of an ITE or canal instrument, or a crack in the shell, itself.

The patient requires more volume when hearing thresholds drop. Feedback from a higher volume will also give indications of other problems:

a. patient uses higher number on volume wheel.

b. hearing instrument analyzer graph at user level shows more gain.

c. ear canal shows redness, wax or infection.

d. patient has cold, sinus, or other medical problem.

e. patient notices unexplained change of hearing.

f. Impedance testing indicates Type C or B tympanograms.

g. audiometric thresholds decrease.
   Adjustments include:

   1. medical referral to correct the medically treatable problems, then reversing adjustments after treatment.

   2. decreasing the vent size.

   3. adding more low frequencies on potentiometer.

   4. using smaller ohm damper, or no damper at all.

   5. replacing the earmold with different acoustic characteristics.

Acoustic feedback sounds like a ringing or vibration before it reaches the squeal stage. A hearing instrument analyzer graph shows sharp peaks between 1500 - 4000 Hz, usually from the receiver. The problem is poor isolation of either or both transducers.

Mechanical feedback has a lower pitched squeal than acoustic feedback. The receiver vibrates the hearing instrument case. Factory repair replaces grommets on transducers.

Magnetic feedback sounds like two microphones too close to each other. Two magnetic fields coupling, like a telephone coil and microphone, or receiver, cause magnetic feedback. Electret microphones have reduced this problem.

Electronic feedback, the good kind of feedback, uses feedback loops, or phase cancelling, like input compression or directional hearing instruments.

Electrostatic feedback sounds like low frequency broad band noise or motorboating. Inadequate decoupling of the battery and amplifier can be corrected by smoother frequency responses, reducing high frequencies, reducing gain, smaller vents, use of dampers and filters, or manufacturer repair. The problem intensifies with a weak battery.

Amplifiers, usually integrated circuits (IC's), capacitors, and resistors, **burn out** with electrical static and corrode with body oils and cosmetics. Pulling sweaters over your head or brushing your hair with the hearing instruments on creates enough static to burn out the instrument. Make it a practice to remind patients of this fact.

Motorboating is usually caused by a build-up of static electricity in the circuit, a weak battery, or corroded battery contacts. Sometimes the manufacturer finds a defective volume control, or burned out capacitor, resistor or amplifier.

Solutions include opening the battery door at night, using a dry-aid kit and wiping moisture or sweat off the battery during the day. The hearing instrument power and clarity fluctuates when the battery shorts out due to moisture.

PROBLEMS with the PATIENT'S VOICE

When ear canal resonance changes with amplification, the patient notices a difference in the quality of their own voice. The change in the perceived quality of the patient's voice can be quite annoying.

The loudest vowel is the 'ah' sound in 'all', and the softest consonant, the 'th' sound in 'thin'. In average speech, the difference between these two sounds is about 28 dB. If you plug your ears, the 'ay' sound, like in play, sounds much louder than 'ah'. Bone conduction and the occlusion effect change the way you hear your voice. A hearing instrument or earmold plugs the ear. The patient only accepts amplification when the sound of their voice is acceptable. Modification is critical to the acceptance of the hearing instrument. Qualify the patient's remarks.

To change ear canal resonance, or shift the resonant frequency upward in frequency you may:

1. enlarge the vent.

2. use an external vent.

3. use slit leak venting by buffing the entire canal surface and tapering the canal tip slightly.

4. shorten the length of the canal.

Most, but not all, voice problems relate to too many low frequencies. **An echo, a vibration, hollow sounds, a plugged feeling, distortion, or feeling like the patient is coming down with a cold,** all describe too much low frequency amplification.

Solutions to reduce lower frequencies include:

a. more airspace in the ear canal. You require a shorter earmold or a larger vent. Use a slit leak vent if venting is not possible.

b. make an acoustic adjustment to tone control potentiometers or use of different dampers.

c. plug the vent from the canal end, rather than the faceplate, to eliminate a 500 Hz resonant cavity.

When the patient complains **that their voice shoots over to their ear or are bothered by certain sounds (like water running)** then check the distance between MCL and UCL. Make sure the patient is not using the hearing instrument gain above the Reference Test Position. The patient requires more range between MCL and UCL. The normal range is greater than the range of the hearing instrument.

The opposite effect of too many lows is too many highs. Patients describe the perception of their voice as being **too tinny, too sharp, or artificial sounding.**

Solutions include:

a. reducing the vent size.

b. lowering the tone controls or changing dampers.

c. tighter fitting earmold.

d. the manufacturer change of microphone or receiver to a lower frequency response.

Low frequency gain is increased when the size of the receiver tubing is reduced or with the use of some type of wax guard

If the patient **'has their head in a barrel',** rather than the sound bouncing or shooting to the ear, or **'feels like they are in a large, empty room', or has an 'echo bouncing**

back at them', the output of the hearing instrument is too high. If you have no output pot, try lamb's wool or a red Knowles filter in the receiver tube or hearing instrument earhook.

When the patient feels their voice is **raspy in their throat,** solutions include:

a. Shortening the tubing if it extends past end of hearing instrument or earmold and vibrates.

b. Turning the hearing instrument louder, patient requires more volume.

c. Filing lower canal area along back and bottom, Vagus nerve pressure creates occlusion effect.

'My chewing is too loud' requires enlarging the vent, shortening the canal, or both.

'My ear feels plugged, like I'm wearing muffs' requires more gain at 1000 Hz area. This may also include 750 Hz and 1500 Hz. Or, they are wearing the hearing instrument too low.

BACKGROUND NOISE

The ability to concentrate on a speaker with noise in the background requires consistent practice. When both ears are impaired, using only one hearing instrument, or only one ear, makes the task more difficult.

Binaural listening situations, with both Maximum Power Output (MPO) and Most Comfortable Level (MCL) balanced, give an improvement in the:

a. signal-to-noise ratio.

b. sense of direction - the noise comes from a different location than the speaker.

c. quieter use levels.

d. binaural summation. The speaker's voice appears louder with both hearing instruments than with a single instrument.

Although binaural listening is preferred, a monaural fitting situation can be improved with:

a. noise switches.

b. higher frequency response.

c. reduced low frequencies - using either tone potentiometers, venting, gain reduction pots.

d. turning down the volume control in noise.

Sometimes, control of background noise requires a circuit change.

People with narrow dynamic ranges, low UCL's, multiple signal processors, often hear better in noise with a plugged vent. All sounds pass through the hearing instrument to reach the eardrum. Loud noise is under the control of the hearing instrument circuit, rather than passing freely through the vent.

COMFORT ADJUSTMENTS

Shell modifications for comfort fall into two categories. If discomfort occurs after wearing the instrument or earmold for a long period, small modifications correct the fit. When discomfort is immediate, greater modification is necessary. Let a sore spot, broken skin, or blister heal before wearing the hearing instrument full time.

Warning - Not all ITE manufacturers honor warranty if you modify the hearing instrument. Consult your manufacturer for permission.

Caution - Plug microphone and/or receiver opening with foam before grinding or buffing to prevent clogging with debris.

ALWAYS use a battery in the hearing instrument, even if the battery is dead. This protects the hearing instrument from static build-up and keeps the circuit polarized during modifications.

LOCATING POINT of DISCOMFORT

Use the otoscope to locate a sore spot in the ear, then match the area on the hearing instrument. Reduce the area on the hearing instrument, opposite the sore spot by grinding and buffing the instrument. For example, when the helix hurts, the intertragal notch is also red. Reducing both of the areas on the hearing instrument allows the instrument to fit properly without pushing the helix up.

When you like the acoustic response of the hearing instrument and need to shorten the canal for comfort, **reduce the size of vent one size for each 1/4" you shorten.** You also reduce overall output by shortening the canal.

GRINDING and BUFFING

A bench grinder can be set up with grinding tools on the right of the motor, and buffing tools on the left, often with two buffing wheels. Buff at low speed. Use one wheel with the buffing compound. Keep the other wheel clean to polish the final shine or finish. Carefully buff thin spots to avoid going through the shell. When in doubt about thin spots, 'candle' the hearing instrument - hold it over a 100 watt bulb. Thin areas are lighter, thicker areas darker. When using buffing and grinding tools you should always wear safety glasses.

REMOVAL NOTCHES

Cut a slit into the faceplate with a small ball burr, or a hand held file. Make the notches accessible to the patient's fingernails at the bottom of the hearing instrument or at the top of the helix area.

DISTORTION

Resonant distortion, sounding like a broken speaker on a radio, occurs when receiver tubing no longer seals entirely to the sound bore. Measurable changes in response, gain and output also occur. As the opening increases, the hearing instrument produces internal feedback.

Intermodulation distortion adds a harshness to speech or music. Sounds are similar to looking in a fun house mirror. Lower frequency sounds are boomy and muffled, high frequencies metalic and harsh. This distortion builds up to create 'listener fatigue.' Intermodulation distortion requires complex sound, so will go undetected with standard test equipment, but not by the human ear. Filters or dampers relieve these the sum and difference frequencies.

Transient distortion sounds like a bang or ringing sound. The ear detects it, but no hearing instrument analyzer using ANSI Standards measure it. This is caused by microphone and receiver inertia, and it clouds the detail of speech or music.

Harmonic distortion depends on the amount of power a hearing instrument produces. The most meaningful measurements are at the patient's volume control settings. 1% is detectable, 3% not objectionable. Harmonic distortion is not as noticable with music as with speech.

CIRCUIT NOISE

Patients may hear circuit noise with:

a. a linear hearing instrument.

b. a high gain, high output hearing instrument.

c. a hearing instrument with mismatched components.

Circuit noise is more prevalent in Automatic Signal Processers (ASP's) circuits.

BODY-WORN HEARING INSTRUMENTS

Body-worn hearing instruments are subject to the same repair problems as other hearing instruments. Because they are worn next to the body, usually in the center or in a shirt pocket, falling food and drinks may plug the microphone opening.

The receiver cord plugs firmly into a jack on the hearing instrument. An intermittent hearing instrument problem may occur with the loose jack connections of the receiver cord into the external receiver or body-worn instrument casing.

A worn cord may produce intermittent difficulty. Twist and roll the receiver cord between your fingers to pinpoint a break in the wire. Perspiration turns the cord green at a break. These spots occur most often near the plug at each end of the cord, or at a point where the cord is pinned to a garment or the patient's hair.

Cord lengths and plugs may differ from model to model, with two prongs, or three prongs. The size of the prongs also differ. When one prong on a two prong cord is larger than the other, the cord is polarized. It only attaches to the hearing instrument one way. If both prongs are the same, the cord can be inserted either way. The cord also attaches firmly to the external receiver, either bone or air conduction. It is a good idea for these patients to carry a spare cord.

A body-worn hearing instrument has less potential for vibration and feedback worn on the opposite side of the body from the ear being fit.

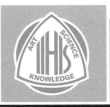
TEST INSTRUCTIONS

After you have finished reading this lesson, carefully study the selections from the **Required Reading.**

Then, look over the lesson once more to impress the important points on your memory.

When you are sure you know the lesson thoroughly, use the answer sheet in the back of the manual that corresponds to this lesson.

IMPORTANT: Place your student number on the answer sheets. Your student number appears on the inside front cover of the manual. **It must appear on your answer sheets in order for you to get credit for completion of the lesson.**

Once the answer sheet is completed, tear it out and mail to: International Institute for Hearing Instruments Studies
16880 Middlebelt Road, Suite 4, Livonia, MI 48154-3367

REQUIRED READING FOR THIS LESSON

Pages 562-583
Hearing Instrument Science and Fitting Practices (Second Edition)

TEST QUESTIONS

1. **The signal/noise ratio of a hearing aid response is:**
    a. the amount of noise a hearing aid makes when an earmold does not fit the ear
    b. of very little significance in fitting a hearing aid
    c. the difference in decibels between the signal and the noise in the system
    d. a comparison of the 90 dB and 60 dB input signals

2. **Acoustic gain is measured in:**
    a. dynes / cm^2
    b. Hertz
    c. decibels SPL
    d. decibels HL

3. **High Frequency Average (HFA) full-on gain is measured by averaging the gain at:**
    a. 500, 1000 and 2000 Hz
    b. 400, 800, and 1600 Hz
    c. 1000, 1600 and 2500 Hz
    d. 2000, 3000 and 4000 Hz

4. **High Frequency Average SSPL 90 (HFA SSPL 90) refers to:**
   a. high frequency average saturation sound pressure level with a 90 dB SPL input
   b. sound pressure level at the maximum frequency
   c. reference test gain
   d. reference test position

5. **The Saturation Sound Pressure level should:**
   a. be between 120 and 130 dB for the average case
   b. be less than 120 dB for tolerance problems
   c. directly relate to the client's UCL
   d. be closer to MCL than UCL

6. **ANSI standards can compare:**
   a. one instrument to another
   b. one kind of loss to another
   c. patient's gain requirements
   d. patient's output requirements

7. **The SSPL90 curve measures:**
   a. all the tones across frequency
   b. the frequency and intensity of the loudest tone only
   c. only the three frequencies necessary for HFA
   d. the intensities of a tone until it saturates at 90 dB

8. **All ANSI instrument measurements are:**
   a. SPL
   b. HL
   c. SL
   d. 0.02 dynes/cm^2

9. **Input sound pressure is measured:**
   a. at the microphone opening of the hearing instrument
   b. at the receiver opening of the hearing instrument
   c. at the microphone of the 2 cc coupler
   d. at the tip of the 2 cc coupler

10. **Gain control is another name for:**
    a. output potentiometer
    b. amplifier
    c. volume wheel
    d. input at the microphone

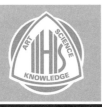
TEST INSTRUCTIONS

After you have finished reading this lesson, carefully study the selections from the **Required Reading.**

Then, look over the lesson once more to impress the important points on your memory.

When you are sure you know the lesson thoroughly, use the answer sheet in the back of the manual that corresponds to this lesson.

IMPORTANT: Place your student number on the answer sheets. Your student number appears on the inside front cover of the manual. **It must appear on your answer sheets in order for you to get credit for completion of the lesson.**

Once the answer sheet is completed, tear it out and mail to: International Institute for Hearing Instruments Studies
16880 Middlebelt Road, Suite 4, Livonia, MI 48154-3367

REQUIRED READING FOR THIS LESSON

Pages 351-429
Hearing Instrument Science and Fitting Practices (Second Edition)

Pages 48-70 – **Outcome Measures & Troubleshooting**

TEST QUESTIONS

1. **A small pressure vent (0.020 to 0.030) in an earmold will:**
    a. have little or no effect on frequencies above 400 Hz
    b. generally reduce levels at frequencies below 200 Hz
    c. reduce atmospheric pressure build-up
    d. all of the above

2. **A long canal on the earmold has the effect of:**
    a. accentuating the low frequencies
    b. increasing the high frequencies
    c. flattening the peaks of the mid-range frequencies
    d. increasing both high and low frequencies without effecting the mid-range

3. **Venting an earmold:**
    a. is necessary in all high gain fittings
    b. should always be used for low frequency losses
    c. is the most common modification made on an earmold
    d. should only be used to relieve a 'plugged' feeling on a new client

4. **The non-occluding earmold is excellent to use on:**
   a. a client with draining ears who does not want to see a physician
   b. a CROS fitting
   c. all cases of bilateral fittings
   d. none of the above

5. **Earmolds have two important parts:**
   a. shell and skeleton
   b. vented and unvented
   c. outer appearance and canal acoustics
   d. hard and soft material

6. **The greatest acoustic change in an earmold or ITE is:**
   a. using dampers
   b. parallel venting
   c. tubing size
   d. outer appearance

7. **The greatest deciding factors in material selection for an earmold are:**
   a. power requirements
   b. the compatibility with dampers
   c. the style of mold
   d. body temperature

8. **To shift the resonant peak upward between 1500-3000 Hz, use:**
   a. smaller ID tubing
   b. smaller OD tubing
   c. larger bore diameter
   d. a longer canal

9. **In general, mold modifications are as follows:**
   a. venting affects lows, damping the midrange and horn effects boost highs
   b. damping affects lows, horn effects boost midrange and venting changes highs
   c. horn modifications change lows, venting changes midrange and dampers affect highs
   d. horn modifications change lows, damping the midrange and venting affects highs

10. **Which molds have the same outer appearance:**
    a. skeleton and 2 HF
    b. standard and shell
    c. half skeleton and half shell
    d. Janssen and Acoustic modifier

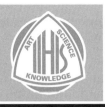

TEST INSTRUCTIONS

After you have finished reading this lesson, carefully study the selections from the **Required Reading.**

Then, look over the lesson once more to impress the important points on your memory.

When you are sure you know the lesson thoroughly, use the answer sheet in the back of the manual that corresponds to this lesson.

IMPORTANT: Place your student number on the answer sheets. Your student number appears on the inside front cover of the manual. **It must appear on your answer sheets in order for you to get credit for completion of the lesson.**

Once the answer sheet is completed, tear it out and mail to: International Institute for Hearing Instruments Studies
16880 Middlebelt Road, Suite 4, Livonia, MI 48154-3367

REQUIRED READING FOR THIS LESSON

Pages 699-710, 741-788
Hearing Instrument Science and Fitting Practices (Second Edition)

TEST QUESTIONS

1. **Residual hearing, in combination with the hearing instrument, will:**
   a. replace or restore hearing to normal
   b. sound natural
   c. help improve communication
   d. allow the patient to adjust to the instrument in just a few days

2. **At night, the battery in the instrument:**
   a. should be removed
   b. can be left in the open battery door
   c. is safe in the instrument as long as the switch is in the 'off' position
   d. should be changed and ready for the next day

3. **A BTE instrument, properly attached:**
   a. fits the contour of the ear
   b. is slightly raised at the bottom of the instrument so the ear, itself, does not get sore
   c. clears the top of the ear slightly to make room for glasses
   d. cannot be worn while using glasses

4. **An advantage of a CIC fitting is:**
   a. improved battery life
   b. reduced acoustic feedback during phone use
   c. decreased wind noise
   d. b and c above

5. **When adjusting the volume control, the patient must:**
   a. find the exact spot where you require use gain
   b. hear quiet speakers in a normal voice
   c. hear loud speakers in a normal voice
   d. find an area on the control where sounds are comfortable

6. **When a standard instrument has a telephone coil, the patient:**
   a. can automatically hear better on the phone
   b. needs to increase the volume control
   c. switches to the 'T' position, then (b) above
   d. has 'feedback' when putting the phone near the instrument

7. **Advise the patient to wear the instrument:**
   a. every other day for two hours
   b. regularly on a daily basis
   c. only when the patient needs to hear
   d. as little as possible to preserve natural hearing

8. **Binaural amplification allows the patient to:**
   a. wear both instruments at a quieter volume setting
   b. wear both instruments at a louder volume setting
   c. hear better, even though they cannot locate the source of the sound
   d. hear better when they tell the speaker to move to the good ear

9. **The patient maintains the instrument by:**
   a. lubricating it weekly
   b. keeping it clean and free of wax
   c. washing it when washing the face or hair
   d. storing it in the 'fridge' with the batteries

10. **Teach the patient to:**
    a. operate the potentiometer settings
    b. operate the OTM switches and noise switches
    c. clean the microphone opening daily
    d. all of the above

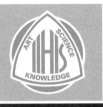
TEST INSTRUCTIONS

After you have finished reading this lesson, carefully study the selections from the **Required Reading.**

Then, look over the lesson once more to impress the important points on your memory.

When you are sure you know the lesson thoroughly, use the answer sheet in the back of the manual that corresponds to this lesson.

IMPORTANT: Place your student number on the answer sheets. Your student number appears on the inside front cover of the manual. **It must appear on your answer sheets in order for you to get credit for completion of the lesson.**

Once the answer sheet is completed, tear it out and mail to: International Institute for Hearing Instruments Studies
16880 Middlebelt Road, Suite 4, Livonia, MI 48154-3367

REQUIRED READING FOR THIS LESSON

Pages 722-739, 597-626, 627-645
Hearing Instrument Science and Fitting Practices (Second Edition)

TEST QUESTIONS

1. **Basic verification involves:**
   a. checking MCL and UCL in quiet and noise
   b. many volume control adjustments
   c. teaching the patient to adjust tone and output potentiometers
   d. instructions on T/C use

2. **Verification procedures:**
   a. check the accuracy of your fitting
   b. do not allow you to adjust or modify effectively
   c. demonstrate the ineffectiveness of restoring the patient to normal
   d. are unnecessary when the patient is a previous user

3. **An effective verification is:**
   a. listening to a watch tick
   b. hearing the words in a song
   c. a measurable improvement in communication
   d. when the patient says he hears better

4. **Functional gain of the instrument:**
   a. is the same as the SSPL90 curve
   b. is at or above RTP
   c. cannot be calculated
   d. is one method of fitting verification

5. **Speech tests measured through the audiometer circuit:**
   a. are 20 dB less because of ANSI Standards
   b. are 20 dB SPL more because of ANSI Standards
   c. need no conversion when in free field
   d. cannot be administered because the headset makes the hearing instrument 'feedback'

6. **Ideally, when presenting recorded words in noise:**
   a. the noise is 10 dB louder than the words
   b. the noise and words are equal in loudness
   c. the words are 10 dB louder than the noise
   d. combined words and noise are 70 dBA or less

7. **Sound field is:**
   a. when sound is either absorbed or dissipated before it strikes a reflected surface
   b. a controlled environment
   c. an anechoic chamber
   d. (a) and (c) above

8. **Most patients use enough gain in the hearing instrument to understand quiet speech at a level of:**
   a. 55 dB SPL
   b. 60 dB SPL
   c. 65 dB SPL
   d. 70 dB SPL

9. **When UCL's are not balanced, a loud signal is perceived as:**
   a. coming from the center of the head
   b. lateralizing to the ear with the higher output
   c. lateralizing to the ear with the lower output
   d. summing into a single hearing experience

10. **The following measurements use SPL as a reference:**
    a. probe microphones
    b. sound field aided thresholds
    c. ANSI specifications
    d. all of the above

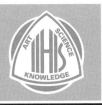

DISTANCE LEARNING for PROFESSIONALS in HEARING HEALTH SCIENCES

Lesson 28 Real Ear Measurement

TEST INSTRUCTIONS

After you have finished reading this lesson, carefully study the selections from the **Required Reading.**

Then, look over the lesson once more to impress the important points on your memory.

When you are sure you know the lesson thoroughly, use the answer sheet in the back of the manual that corresponds to this lesson.

IMPORTANT: Place your student number on the answer sheets. Your student number appears on the inside front cover of the manual. **It must appear on your answer sheets in order for you to get credit for completion of the lesson.**

Once the answer sheet is completed, tear it out and mail to: International Institute for Hearing Instruments Studies
16880 Middlebelt Road, Suite 4, Livonia, MI 48154-3367

REQUIRED READING FOR THIS LESSON

Pages 627-643
Hearing Instrument Science and Fitting Practices (Second Edition)

Pages 2-29
Outcome Measures & Troubleshooting

TEST QUESTIONS

1. **Which of the following is not a coupler used for measuring hearing aid performance:**
   a. Zwisks Ear Simulator
   b. the human ear
   c. 2cc Hard Walled coupler
   d. Knowles Electronic Manikin for Acoustic Response

2. **A Real Ear Measurement System incorporates all of the following:**
   a. Signal Generator, Reference Microphone, Measurement Microphone, Display Device
   b. Signal Enhancer, Computer, Measurement Microphone, Speaker
   c. Display Device, Reference Microphone, 2cc Coupler, Probe Tube
   d. Computer, Reference Microphone, Speaker, Graphic Equalizer

3. **REUR Measurements are taken in:**
   a. an open human ear canal
   b. 2cc hard walled coupler
   c. an ear canal with a hearing aid inserted and turned on
   d. an open ear canal on KEMAR

4. **At what distance from the Tympanic Membrane should the end of the probe tube be placed:**
   a. Within 5 millimeters
   b. Even with the end of the earmold
   c. 10 millimeters from the end of the earmold
   d. Touching the TM

5. **When testing compression hearing aids which signal type is best to use:**
   a. Fast Fourier Transform
   b. Swept Pure Tones
   c. 70dB
   d. NAL-R

6. **Loud speaker placement should be:**
   a. 1 meter at 45° azimuth
   b. 1.5 meters at 90° azimuth
   c. .5 meters at 0° azimuth
   d. Does not make any difference

7. **Which of the following is not included in correct test protocols:**
   a. Plugging the hearing aid vent to control feedback
   b. Adjusting the Probe Tube to minimize Standing Waves
   c. Using the same stimulus type and level for all measurements
   d. Inserting the instrument with the power turned off

8. **RESR Measurements for compression hearing aids have been replaced with:**
   a. A family of curves starting at a soft level and gradually increasing in intensity
   b. SSPL-90 curves in a test box
   c. Real Ear Aided Responses
   d. SSPL-90 curves on KEMAR

9. **Which of he following Real Ear Targets has been documented to be the best for Non-Linear Hearing Aids:**
   a. None have been proven to be better than any other
   b. NAL-Revised
   c. DSL(I/O)
   d. IHAFF

10. **Insertion Loss occurs when:**
    a. The level in the ear canal with a hearing aid inserted is less than the input level
    b. The level in the ear canal with a hearing aid inserted is greater than the input level
    c. Rarely happens during REOR measurements
    d. Is an artifact of the sound field

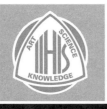

TEST INSTRUCTIONS

After you have finished reading this lesson, carefully study the selections from the **Required Reading.**

Then, look over the lesson once more to impress the important points on your memory.

When you are sure you know the lesson thoroughly, use the answer sheet in the back of the manual that corresponds to this lesson.

IMPORTANT: Place your student number on the answer sheets. Your student number appears on the inside front cover of the manual. **It must appear on your answer sheets in order for you to get credit for completion of the lesson.**

Once the answer sheet is completed, tear it out and mail to: International Institute for Hearing Instruments Studies
16880 Middlebelt Road, Suite 4, Livonia, MI 48154-3367

REQUIRED READING FOR THIS LESSON

Pages 710-739, 836-840
Hearing Instrument Science and Fitting Practices (Second Edition)
Pages 1 - 50
Altering Behaviors

TEST QUESTIONS

1. **Follow-up care is a variety of procedures which comprise:**
   a. long term management of the client's needs and use of amplification
   b. a process which never ends while the client is under the care of the hearing aid specialist
   c. bringing out the best that the instrument can give
   d. all of the above

2. **Emphasizing counseling to maximize amplification benefits is:**
   a. a new technique
   b. a program that should start before the fitting
   c. beneficial to only a few
   d. not within the scope of the hearing aid specialist's responsibilities

3. **Aural rehabilitation:**
   a. is unnecessary for previous users
   b. only involves the patient during the fitting
   c. produces unreasonable expectations
   d. continues for as long as the patient wears an instrument

4. **Patients are always aware of:**
   a. impacted wax
   b. hard earmold tubing
   c. corroded battery contacts
   d. the way they hear today

5. **When the patient experiences difficulties, one of the problems could be:**
   a. a procedural flaw in the original hearing loss assessment
   b. an error in judgement in hearing instrument selection
   c. misestimation of some aspect of the hearing problem
   d. all of the above

6. **User satisfaction must include:**
   a. optimal acoustic response
   b. patient preference
   c. best aided response
   d. best instrument for noisy environments

7. **Client acceptance involves counseling on:**
   a. personal family problems
   b. emotional and social concerns
   c. attitude and motivation
   d. (b) and (c) above

8. **Friends and family help patients wearing hearing instruments to hear better by:**
   a. talking louder, close to the ear
   b. sitting the patient in the middle of the room
   c. encouraging the patient to have a light behind them
   d. combining visual clues

9. **Your counseling avoids:**
   a. unreasonable expectations
   b. using visual clues
   c. service reminders
   d. the use of counsellors, special workers and psychologists

10. **Family and friends can have a negative influence on the patient by:**
    a. showing the patient how to handle the instrument
    b. expressing frustration that the patient does not have 'normal' hearing
    c. helping the patient to insert the instrument
    d. encouraging instrument use

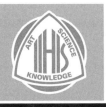
TEST INSTRUCTIONS

After you have finished reading this lesson, carefully study the selections from the **Required Reading.**

Then, look over the lesson once more to impress the important points on your memory.

When you are sure you know the lesson thoroughly, use the answer sheet in the back of the manual that corresponds to this lesson.

IMPORTANT: Place your student number on the answer sheets. Your student number appears on the inside front cover of the manual. **It must appear on your answer sheets in order for you to get credit for completion of the lesson.**

Once the answer sheet is completed, tear it out and mail to: International Institute for Hearing Instruments Studies
16880 Middlebelt Road, Suite 4, Livonia, MI 48154-3367

REQUIRED READING FOR THIS LESSON

Pages 271-281, 415-425
Hearing Instrument Science and Fitting Practices (Second Edition)

TEST QUESTIONS

1. **When a hearing aid sounds weak, hollow, distorted, or intermittent, the first check is:**
   a. a plugged receiver
   b. faulty volume control
   c. a weak battery
   d. broken microphone wire

2. **An otoscope helps when cleaning the:**
   a. microphone
   b. receiver
   c. earhook
   d. earmold

3. **When a hearing aid is dead, you can check receiver and microphone function by:**
   a. turning the instrument to telecoil
   b. advancing the volume control to full on with the instrument on 'M'
   c. opening the battery door to see if you hear a 'click'
   d. cleaning the receiver with a wax loop

4. **A hearing aid that works with the battery door slightly open, but shuts off when you close the door has:**
   a. wires touching the battery
   b. a broken microphone wire
   c. a faulty volume control
   d. a weak battery

5. **You CANNOT use feedback checks when:**
   a. adjusting a tone pot
   b. adjusting an output pot
   c. checking volume control intermittency
   d. checking the telephone coil

6. **An earhook damper is plugged when, during a feedback check:**
   a. feedback remains unchanged with volume control rotation
   b. feedback occurs only with the volume control at MAX
   c. the instrument makes no sound during any test
   d. the instrument feeds back only when the coupler is removed

7. **A sign of a dirty volume control is:**
   a. the instrument is dead
   b. constant feedback
   c. intermittent static
   d. motorboating

8. **Reduction of background noise can be improved by:**
   a. using a windscreen
   b. reducing tubing size
   c. directional microphones
   d. none of the above

9. **When a new hearing instrument has feedback at the patient's comfortable level, the problem is usually:**
   a. too much wax in the ear canal
   b. smaller vent than appropriate
   c. manufacturer's error
   d. split receiver tubing

10. **An ITE or Canal aid has internal feedback when:**
    a. the receiver tubing has excess wax
    b. the receiver tubing is not completely sealed to the sound bore
    c. the vent size is too large
    d. the patient loses weight

INTERNATIONAL INSTITUTE FOR HEARING INSTRUMENTS STUDIES

DISTANCE LEARNING for Professionals in HEARING HEALTH SCIENCES

THE OUTER EAR

LESSON 1

FIFTH EDITION

STUDENT NUMBER

◀ Enter your five digit student number found on the inside front cover of this manual into the box at left.

■ Completely fill in the circle that indicates the correct answer.

■ Upon completion, tear out the answer sheet and return it for scoring to: IIHIS, 16880 Middlebelt Road, Suite 4, Livonia, MI 48154-3367

1. Ⓐ Ⓑ Ⓒ Ⓓ

2. Ⓐ Ⓑ Ⓒ Ⓓ

3. Ⓐ Ⓑ Ⓒ Ⓓ

4. Ⓐ Ⓑ Ⓒ Ⓓ

5. Ⓐ Ⓑ Ⓒ Ⓓ

6. Ⓐ Ⓑ Ⓒ Ⓓ

7. Ⓐ Ⓑ Ⓒ Ⓓ

OFFICE USE ONLY

DATE RECEIVED

/ /

8. Ⓐ Ⓑ Ⓒ Ⓓ

GRADE

9. Ⓐ Ⓑ Ⓒ Ⓓ

10. Ⓐ Ⓑ Ⓒ Ⓓ

IIHIS   ANSWER SHEET

INTERNATIONAL INSTITUTE FOR HEARING INSTRUMENTS STUDIES

DISTANCE LEARNING for Professionals in HEARING HEALTH SCIENCES

DISORDERS OF THE OUTER EAR

LESSON 2

FIFTH EDITION

STUDENT NUMBER

◀ Enter your five digit student number found on the inside front cover of this manual into the box at left.

- Completely fill in the circle that indicates the correct answer.

- Upon completion, tear out the answer sheet and return it for scoring to: IIHIS, 16880 Middlebelt Road, Suite 4, Livonia, MI 48154-3367

1. (A) (B) (C) (D)

2. (A) (B) (C) (D)

3. (A) (B) (C) (D)

4. (A) (B) (C) (D)

5. (A) (B) (C) (D)

6. (A) (B) (C) (D)

7. (A) (B) (C) (D)

8. (A) (B) (C) (D)

9. (A) (B) (C) (D)

10. (A) (B) (C) (D)

INTERNATIONAL INSTITUTE FOR HEARING INSTRUMENTS STUDIES

DISTANCE LEARNING for Professionals in HEARING HEALTH SCIENCES

THE MIDDLE EAR OR TYMPANIC CAVITY

LESSON 3

FIFTH EDITION

STUDENT NUMBER

◀ Enter your five digit student number found on the inside front cover of this manual into the box at left.

■ Completely fill in the circle that indicates the correct answer.

■ Upon completion, tear out the answer sheet and return it for scoring to: IIHIS, 16880 Middlebelt Road, Suite 4, Livonia, MI 48154-3367

1. Ⓐ Ⓑ Ⓒ Ⓓ

2. Ⓐ Ⓑ Ⓒ Ⓓ

3. Ⓐ Ⓑ Ⓒ Ⓓ

4. Ⓐ Ⓑ Ⓒ Ⓓ

5. Ⓐ Ⓑ Ⓒ Ⓓ

6. Ⓐ Ⓑ Ⓒ Ⓓ

7. Ⓐ Ⓑ Ⓒ Ⓓ

8. Ⓐ Ⓑ Ⓒ Ⓓ

9. Ⓐ Ⓑ Ⓒ Ⓓ

10. Ⓐ Ⓑ Ⓒ Ⓓ

OFFICE USE ONLY

DATE RECEIVED

/ /

GRADE

IIHIS

A N S W E R   S H E E T

INTERNATIONAL INSTITUTE FOR HEARING INSTRUMENTS STUDIES

DISTANCE LEARNING for Professionals in HEARING HEALTH SCIENCES

DISORDERS OF THE MIDDLE EAR

LESSON 4

FIFTH EDITION

STUDENT NUMBER

◀ Enter your five digit student number found on the inside front cover of this manual into the box at left.

■ Completely fill in the circle that indicates the correct answer.

■ Upon completion, tear out the answer sheet and return it for scoring to: IIHIS, 16880 Middlebelt Road, Suite 4, Livonia, MI 48154-3367

1. Ⓐ Ⓑ Ⓒ Ⓓ

2. Ⓐ Ⓑ Ⓒ Ⓓ

3. Ⓐ Ⓑ Ⓒ Ⓓ

4. Ⓐ Ⓑ Ⓒ Ⓓ

5. Ⓐ Ⓑ Ⓒ Ⓓ

6. Ⓐ Ⓑ Ⓒ Ⓓ

7. Ⓐ Ⓑ Ⓒ Ⓓ

OFFICE USE ONLY

DATE RECEIVED

/   /

8. Ⓐ Ⓑ Ⓒ Ⓓ

GRADE

9. Ⓐ Ⓑ Ⓒ Ⓓ

10. Ⓐ Ⓑ Ⓒ Ⓓ

IIHIS   **A N S W E R   S H E E T**

INTERNATIONAL INSTITUTE FOR HEARING INSTRUMENTS STUDIES

DISTANCE LEARNING for Professionals in HEARING HEALTH SCIENCES

THE INNER EAR & AUDITORY PATHWAYS

LESSON 5

FIFTH EDITION

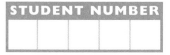

STUDENT NUMBER

◀ Enter your five digit student number found on the inside front cover of this manual into the box at left.

■ Completely fill in the circle that indicates the correct answer.

■ Upon completion, tear out the answer sheet and return it for scoring to: IIHIS, 16880 Middlebelt Road, Suite 4, Livonia, MI 48154-3367

1. Ⓐ Ⓑ Ⓒ Ⓓ

2. Ⓐ Ⓑ Ⓒ Ⓓ

3. Ⓐ Ⓑ Ⓒ Ⓓ

4. Ⓐ Ⓑ Ⓒ Ⓓ

5. Ⓐ Ⓑ Ⓒ Ⓓ

6. Ⓐ Ⓑ Ⓒ Ⓓ

7. Ⓐ Ⓑ Ⓒ Ⓓ

8. Ⓐ Ⓑ Ⓒ Ⓓ

9. Ⓐ Ⓑ Ⓒ Ⓓ

10. Ⓐ Ⓑ Ⓒ Ⓓ

OFFICE USE ONLY

DATE RECEIVED

/ /

GRADE

INTERNATIONAL INSTITUTE FOR HEARING INSTRUMENTS STUDIES

DISTANCE LEARNING for Professionals in HEARING HEALTH SCIENCES

COCHLEAR & RETROCOCHLEAR DISORDERS

LESSON 6

FIFTH EDITION

STUDENT NUMBER

◀ Enter your five digit student number found on the inside front cover of this manual into the box at left.

■ Completely fill in the circle that indicates the correct answer.

■ Upon completion, tear out the answer sheet and return it for scoring to: IIHIS, 16880 Middlebelt Road, Suite 4, Livonia, MI 48154-3367

1. Ⓐ Ⓑ Ⓒ Ⓓ

2. Ⓐ Ⓑ Ⓒ Ⓓ

3. Ⓐ Ⓑ Ⓒ Ⓓ

4. Ⓐ Ⓑ Ⓒ Ⓓ

5. Ⓐ Ⓑ Ⓒ Ⓓ

6. Ⓐ Ⓑ Ⓒ Ⓓ

7. Ⓐ Ⓑ Ⓒ Ⓓ

8. Ⓐ Ⓑ Ⓒ Ⓓ

9. Ⓐ Ⓑ Ⓒ Ⓓ

10. Ⓐ Ⓑ Ⓒ Ⓓ

OFFICE USE ONLY

DATE RECEIVED

/ /

GRADE

IIHIS

ANSWER SHEET

INTERNATIONAL INSTITUTE FOR HEARING INSTRUMENTS STUDIES

DISTANCE LEARNING for Professionals in HEARING HEALTH SCIENCES

INTRODUCTION TO AUDIOMETRY

LESSON 7

FIFTH EDITION

STUDENT NUMBER

◄ Enter your five digit student number found on the inside front cover of this manual into the box at left.

■ Completely fill in the circle that indicates the correct answer.

■ Upon completion, tear out the answer sheet and return it for scoring to: IIHIS, 16880 Middlebelt Road, Suite 4, Livonia, MI 48154-3367

1. Ⓐ Ⓑ Ⓒ Ⓓ

2. Ⓐ Ⓑ Ⓒ Ⓓ

3. Ⓐ Ⓑ Ⓒ Ⓓ

4. Ⓐ Ⓑ Ⓒ Ⓓ

5. Ⓐ Ⓑ Ⓒ Ⓓ

6. Ⓐ Ⓑ Ⓒ Ⓓ

7. Ⓐ Ⓑ Ⓒ Ⓓ

OFFICE USE ONLY

DATE RECEIVED

/ /

8. Ⓐ Ⓑ Ⓒ Ⓓ

GRADE

9. Ⓐ Ⓑ Ⓒ Ⓓ

10. Ⓐ Ⓑ Ⓒ Ⓓ

IIHIS   **A N S W E R   S H E E T**

INTERNATIONAL INSTITUTE FOR HEARING INSTRUMENTS STUDIES

DISTANCE LEARNING for Professionals in HEARING HEALTH SCIENCES

PURE TONE TESTING

LESSON 8

FIFTH EDITION

STUDENT NUMBER

◀ Enter your five digit student number found on the inside front cover of this manual into the box at left.

■ Completely fill in the circle that indicates the correct answer.

■ Upon completion, tear out the answer sheet and return it for scoring to: IIHIS, 16880 Middlebelt Road, Suite 4, Livonia, MI 48154-3367

1. Ⓐ Ⓑ Ⓒ Ⓓ

2. Ⓐ Ⓑ Ⓒ Ⓓ

3. Ⓐ Ⓑ Ⓒ Ⓓ

4. Ⓐ Ⓑ Ⓒ Ⓓ

5. Ⓐ Ⓑ Ⓒ Ⓓ

6. Ⓐ Ⓑ Ⓒ Ⓓ

7. Ⓐ Ⓑ Ⓒ Ⓓ

8. Ⓐ Ⓑ Ⓒ Ⓓ

9. Ⓐ Ⓑ Ⓒ Ⓓ

10. Ⓐ Ⓑ Ⓒ Ⓓ

OFFICE USE ONLY

DATE RECEIVED

/ /

GRADE

INTERNATIONAL INSTITUTE FOR HEARING INSTRUMENTS STUDIES

DISTANCE LEARNING for Professionals in HEARING HEALTH SCIENCES

PURE TONE BONE CONDUCTION TESTS

LESSON 9

FIFTH EDITION

STUDENT NUMBER

◀ Enter your five digit student number found on the inside front cover of this manual into the box at left.

■ Completely fill in the circle that indicates the correct answer.

■ Upon completion, tear out the answer sheet and return it for scoring to: IIHIS, 16880 Middlebelt Road, Suite 4, Livonia, MI 48154-3367

1. Ⓐ Ⓑ Ⓒ Ⓓ

2. Ⓐ Ⓑ Ⓒ Ⓓ

3. Ⓐ Ⓑ Ⓒ Ⓓ

4. Ⓐ Ⓑ Ⓒ Ⓓ

5. Ⓐ Ⓑ Ⓒ Ⓓ

6. Ⓐ Ⓑ Ⓒ Ⓓ

7. Ⓐ Ⓑ Ⓒ Ⓓ

8. Ⓐ Ⓑ Ⓒ Ⓓ

9. Ⓐ Ⓑ Ⓒ Ⓓ

10. Ⓐ Ⓑ Ⓒ Ⓓ

OFFICE USE ONLY

DATE RECEIVED

/ /

GRADE

IIHIS A N S W E R   S H E E T

INTERNATIONAL INSTITUTE FOR HEARING INSTRUMENTS STUDIES

DISTANCE LEARNING for Professionals in HEARING HEALTH SCIENCES

MASKING - PURE TONES

LESSON 10

FIFTH EDITION

STUDENT NUMBER

◀ Enter your five digit student number found on the inside front cover of this manual into the box at left.

■ Completely fill in the circle that indicates the correct answer.

■ Upon completion, tear out the answer sheet and return it for scoring to: IIHIS, 16880 Middlebelt Road, Suite 4, Livonia, MI 48154-3367

1. Ⓐ Ⓑ Ⓒ Ⓓ

2. Ⓐ Ⓑ Ⓒ Ⓓ

3. Ⓐ Ⓑ Ⓒ Ⓓ

4. Ⓐ Ⓑ Ⓒ Ⓓ

5. Ⓐ Ⓑ Ⓒ Ⓓ

6. Ⓐ Ⓑ Ⓒ Ⓓ

7. Ⓐ Ⓑ Ⓒ Ⓓ

8. Ⓐ Ⓑ Ⓒ Ⓓ

9. Ⓐ Ⓑ Ⓒ Ⓓ

10. Ⓐ Ⓑ Ⓒ Ⓓ

INTERNATIONAL INSTITUTE FOR HEARING INSTRUMENTS STUDIES

DISTANCE LEARNING for Professionals in HEARING HEALTH SCIENCES

THE HEARING ANALYSIS: THE AUDIOGRAM

LESSON II

FIFTH EDITION

STUDENT NUMBER

◀ Enter your five digit student number found on the inside front cover of this manual into the box at left.

■ Completely fill in the circle that indicates the correct answer.

■ Upon completion, tear out the answer sheet and return it for scoring to: IIHIS, 16880 Middlebelt Road, Suite 4, Livonia, MI 48154-3367

1. Ⓐ Ⓑ Ⓒ Ⓓ

2. Ⓐ Ⓑ Ⓒ Ⓓ

3. Ⓐ Ⓑ Ⓒ Ⓓ

4. Ⓐ Ⓑ Ⓒ Ⓓ

5. Ⓐ Ⓑ Ⓒ Ⓓ

6. Ⓐ Ⓑ Ⓒ Ⓓ

7. Ⓐ Ⓑ Ⓒ Ⓓ

OFFICE USE ONLY

DATE RECEIVED

/ /

8. Ⓐ Ⓑ Ⓒ Ⓓ

9. Ⓐ Ⓑ Ⓒ Ⓓ

GRADE

10. Ⓐ Ⓑ Ⓒ Ⓓ

IIHIS   **A N S W E R   S H E E T**

INTERNATIONAL INSTITUTE FOR HEARING INSTRUMENTS STUDIES

DISTANCE LEARNING
for Professionals in
HEARING HEALTH SCIENCES

SPEECH TESTING

LESSON 12

FIFTH EDITION

STUDENT NUMBER

◀ Enter your five digit student number found on the inside front cover of this manual into the box at left.

- Completely fill in the circle that indicates the correct answer.

- Upon completion, tear out the answer sheet and return it for scoring to: IIHIS, 16880 Middlebelt Road, Suite 4, Livonia, MI 48154-3367

1. Ⓐ Ⓑ Ⓒ Ⓓ

2. Ⓐ Ⓑ Ⓒ Ⓓ

3. Ⓐ Ⓑ Ⓒ Ⓓ

4. Ⓐ Ⓑ Ⓒ Ⓓ

5. Ⓐ Ⓑ Ⓒ Ⓓ

6. Ⓐ Ⓑ Ⓒ Ⓓ

7. Ⓐ Ⓑ Ⓒ Ⓓ

8. Ⓐ Ⓑ Ⓒ Ⓓ

9. Ⓐ Ⓑ Ⓒ Ⓓ

10. Ⓐ Ⓑ Ⓒ Ⓓ

OFFICE USE ONLY

DATE RECEIVED

/ /

GRADE

IIHIS ANSWER SHEET

INTERNATIONAL INSTITUTE FOR HEARING INSTRUMENTS STUDIES

DISTANCE LEARNING for Professionals in HEARING HEALTH SCIENCES

SPEECH DISCRIMINATION TESTS

LESSON 13

FIFTH EDITION

STUDENT NUMBER

◀ Enter your five digit student number found on the inside front cover of this manual into the box at left.

■ Completely fill in the circle that indicates the correct answer.

■ Upon completion, tear out the answer sheet and return it for scoring to: IIHIS, 16880 Middlebelt Road, Suite 4, Livonia, MI 48154-3367

1. (A) (B) (C) (D)

2. (A) (B) (C) (D)

3. (A) (B) (C) (D)

4. (A) (B) (C) (D)

5. (A) (B) (C) (D)

6. (A) (B) (C) (D)

7. (A) (B) (C) (D)

8. (A) (B) (C) (D)

9. (A) (B) (C) (D)

10. (A) (B) (C) (D)

OFFICE USE ONLY

DATE RECEIVED

/ /

GRADE

IIHIS

A N S W E R   S H E E T

INTERNATIONAL INSTITUTE FOR HEARING INSTRUMENTS STUDIES

DISTANCE LEARNING for Professionals in HEARING HEALTH SCIENCES

TYMPANOMETRY

LESSON 14

FIFTH EDITION

STUDENT NUMBER

◀ Enter your five digit student number found on the inside front cover of this manual into the box at left.

■ Completely fill in the circle that indicates the correct answer.

■ Upon completion, tear out the answer sheet and return it for scoring to: IIHIS, 16880 Middlebelt Road, Suite 4, Livonia, MI 48154-3367

1. Ⓐ Ⓑ Ⓒ Ⓓ

2. Ⓐ Ⓑ Ⓒ Ⓓ

3. Ⓐ Ⓑ Ⓒ Ⓓ

4. Ⓐ Ⓑ Ⓒ Ⓓ

5. Ⓐ Ⓑ Ⓒ Ⓓ

6. Ⓐ Ⓑ Ⓒ Ⓓ

7. Ⓐ Ⓑ Ⓒ Ⓓ

OFFICE USE ONLY

DATE RECEIVED

/ /

GRADE

8. Ⓐ Ⓑ Ⓒ Ⓓ

9. Ⓐ Ⓑ Ⓒ Ⓓ

10. Ⓐ Ⓑ Ⓒ Ⓓ

IIHIS   **A N S W E R   S H E E T**

INTERNATIONAL INSTITUTE FOR HEARING INSTRUMENTS STUDIES

DISTANCE LEARNING for Professionals in HEARING HEALTH SCIENCES

PHYSIOLOGICAL ACOUSTICS

LESSON 15

FIFTH EDITION

STUDENT NUMBER

◀ Enter your five digit student number found on the inside front cover of this manual into the box at left.

■ Completely fill in the circle that indicates the correct answer.

■ Upon completion, tear out the answer sheet and return it for scoring to: IIHIS, 16880 Middlebelt Road, Suite 4, Livonia, MI 48154-3367

1. Ⓐ Ⓑ Ⓒ Ⓓ

2. Ⓐ Ⓑ Ⓒ Ⓓ

3. Ⓐ Ⓑ Ⓒ Ⓓ

4. Ⓐ Ⓑ Ⓒ Ⓓ

5. Ⓐ Ⓑ Ⓒ Ⓓ

6. Ⓐ Ⓑ Ⓒ Ⓓ

7. Ⓐ Ⓑ Ⓒ Ⓓ

8. Ⓐ Ⓑ Ⓒ Ⓓ

9. Ⓐ Ⓑ Ⓒ Ⓓ

10. Ⓐ Ⓑ Ⓒ Ⓓ

INTERNATIONAL INSTITUTE FOR HEARING INSTRUMENTS STUDIES

DISTANCE LEARNING for Professionals in HEARING HEALTH SCIENCES

PSYCHOLOGICAL ACOUSTICS

LESSON 16

FIFTH EDITION

STUDENT NUMBER

◀ Enter your five digit student number found on the inside front cover of this manual into the box at left.

▪ Completely fill in the circle that indicates the correct answer.

▪ Upon completion, tear out the answer sheet and return it for scoring to: IIHIS, 16880 Middlebelt Road, Suite 4, Livonia, MI 48154-3367

1. Ⓐ Ⓑ Ⓒ Ⓓ

2. Ⓐ Ⓑ Ⓒ Ⓓ

3. Ⓐ Ⓑ Ⓒ Ⓓ

4. Ⓐ Ⓑ Ⓒ Ⓓ

5. Ⓐ Ⓑ Ⓒ Ⓓ

6. Ⓐ Ⓑ Ⓒ Ⓓ

7. Ⓐ Ⓑ Ⓒ Ⓓ

8. Ⓐ Ⓑ Ⓒ Ⓓ

9. Ⓐ Ⓑ Ⓒ Ⓓ

10. Ⓐ Ⓑ Ⓒ Ⓓ

OFFICE USE ONLY

DATE RECEIVED

/ /

GRADE

IIHIS

A N S W E R   S H E E T

INTERNATIONAL INSTITUTE FOR HEARING INSTRUMENTS STUDIES

DISTANCE LEARNING for Professionals in HEARING HEALTH SCIENCES

HEARING INSTRUMENT CANDIDACY

LESSON 17

FIFTH EDITION

STUDENT NUMBER

◄ Enter your five digit student number found on the inside front cover of this manual into the box at left.

■ Completely fill in the circle that indicates the correct answer.

■ Upon completion, tear out the answer sheet and return it for scoring to: IIHIS, 16880 Middlebelt Road, Suite 4, Livonia, MI 48154-3367

1. Ⓐ   Ⓑ   Ⓒ   Ⓓ

2. Ⓐ   Ⓑ   Ⓒ   Ⓓ

3. Ⓐ   Ⓑ   Ⓒ   Ⓓ

4. Ⓐ   Ⓑ   Ⓒ   Ⓓ

5. Ⓐ   Ⓑ   Ⓒ   Ⓓ

6. Ⓐ   Ⓑ   Ⓒ   Ⓓ

7. Ⓐ   Ⓑ   Ⓒ   Ⓓ

8. Ⓐ   Ⓑ   Ⓒ   Ⓓ

9. Ⓐ   Ⓑ   Ⓒ   Ⓓ

10. Ⓐ   Ⓑ   Ⓒ   Ⓓ

IIHIS

ANSWER SHEET

INTERNATIONAL INSTITUTE FOR HEARING INSTRUMENTS STUDIES

DISTANCE LEARNING for Professionals in HEARING HEALTH SCIENCES

RATIONALE FOR CIC FITTINGS

LESSON 18

FIFTH EDITION

STUDENT NUMBER

◄ Enter your five digit student number found on the inside front cover of this manual into the box at left.

■ Completely fill in the circle that indicates the correct answer.

■ Upon completion, tear out the answer sheet and return it for scoring to: IIHIS, 16880 Middlebelt Road, Suite 4, Livonia, MI 48154-3367

1. Ⓐ Ⓑ Ⓒ Ⓓ

2. Ⓐ Ⓑ Ⓒ Ⓓ

3. Ⓐ Ⓑ Ⓒ Ⓓ

4. Ⓐ Ⓑ Ⓒ Ⓓ

5. Ⓐ Ⓑ Ⓒ Ⓓ

6. Ⓐ Ⓑ Ⓒ Ⓓ

7. Ⓐ Ⓑ Ⓒ Ⓓ

8. Ⓐ Ⓑ Ⓒ Ⓓ

9. Ⓐ Ⓑ Ⓒ Ⓓ

10. Ⓐ Ⓑ Ⓒ Ⓓ

INTERNATIONAL INSTITUTE FOR HEARING INSTRUMENTS STUDIES

DISTANCE LEARNING for Professionals in HEARING HEALTH SCIENCES

HEARING INSTRUMENTS / DIGITAL TECHNOLOGY

LESSON 19

FIFTH EDITION

STUDENT NUMBER

◀ Enter your five digit student number found on the inside front cover of this manual into the box at left.

■ Completely fill in the circle that indicates the correct answer.

■ Upon completion, tear out the answer sheet and return it for scoring to: IIHIS, 16880 Middlebelt Road, Suite 4, Livonia, MI 48154-3367

1. Ⓐ Ⓑ Ⓒ Ⓓ

2. Ⓐ Ⓑ Ⓒ Ⓓ

3. Ⓐ Ⓑ Ⓒ Ⓓ

4. Ⓐ Ⓑ Ⓒ Ⓓ

5. Ⓐ Ⓑ Ⓒ Ⓓ

6. Ⓐ Ⓑ Ⓒ Ⓓ

7. Ⓐ Ⓑ Ⓒ Ⓓ

8. Ⓐ Ⓑ Ⓒ Ⓓ

9. Ⓐ Ⓑ Ⓒ Ⓓ

10. Ⓐ Ⓑ Ⓒ Ⓓ

OFFICE USE ONLY

DATE RECEIVED

/ /

GRADE

IIHIS   **ANSWER SHEET**

INTERNATIONAL INSTITUTE FOR HEARING INSTRUMENTS STUDIES

DISTANCE LEARNING for Professionals in HEARING HEALTH SCIENCES

OPEN-FIT AND SEALED-FIT MINI BTE HEARING AIDS

LESSON 20

FIFTH EDITION

STUDENT NUMBER

◀ Enter your five digit student number found on the inside front cover of this manual into the box at left.

■ Completely fill in the circle that indicates the correct answer.

■ Upon completion, tear out the answer sheet and return it for scoring to: IIHIS, 16880 Middlebelt Road, Suite 4, Livonia, MI 48154-3367

1. Ⓐ Ⓑ Ⓒ Ⓓ

2. Ⓐ Ⓑ Ⓒ Ⓓ

3. Ⓐ Ⓑ Ⓒ Ⓓ

4. Ⓐ Ⓑ Ⓒ Ⓓ

5. Ⓐ Ⓑ Ⓒ Ⓓ

6. Ⓐ Ⓑ Ⓒ Ⓓ

7. Ⓐ Ⓑ Ⓒ Ⓓ

OFFICE USE ONLY

DATE RECEIVED

/   /

8. Ⓐ Ⓑ Ⓒ Ⓓ

GRADE

9. Ⓐ Ⓑ Ⓒ Ⓓ

10. Ⓐ Ⓑ Ⓒ Ⓓ

IIHIS   **A N S W E R   S H E E T**

INTERNATIONAL INSTITUTE FOR HEARING INSTRUMENTS STUDIES

DISTANCE LEARNING for Professionals in HEARING HEALTH SCIENCES

HEARING INSTRUMENT HISTORY

LESSON 21

FIFTH EDITION

STUDENT NUMBER

◀ Enter your five digit student number found on the inside front cover of this manual into the box at left.

■ Completely fill in the circle that indicates the correct answer.

■ Upon completion, tear out the answer sheet and return it for scoring to: IIHIS, 16880 Middlebelt Road, Suite 4, Livonia, MI 48154-3367

1. Ⓐ Ⓑ Ⓒ Ⓓ

2. Ⓐ Ⓑ Ⓒ Ⓓ

3. Ⓐ Ⓑ Ⓒ Ⓓ

4. Ⓐ Ⓑ Ⓒ Ⓓ

5. Ⓐ Ⓑ Ⓒ Ⓓ

6. Ⓐ Ⓑ Ⓒ Ⓓ

7. Ⓐ Ⓑ Ⓒ Ⓓ

8. Ⓐ Ⓑ Ⓒ Ⓓ

9. Ⓐ Ⓑ Ⓒ Ⓓ

10. Ⓐ Ⓑ Ⓒ Ⓓ

OFFICE USE ONLY

DATE RECEIVED

/ /

GRADE

INTERNATIONAL INSTITUTE FOR HEARING INSTRUMENTS STUDIES

DISTANCE LEARNING for Professionals in HEARING HEALTH SCIENCES

HEARING INSTRUMENT ELECTRONICS

LESSON 22

FIFTH EDITION

STUDENT NUMBER

◀ Enter your five digit student number found on the inside front cover of this manual into the box at left.

■ Completely fill in the circle that indicates the correct answer.

■ Upon completion, tear out the answer sheet and return it for scoring to: IIHIS, 16880 Middlebelt Road, Suite 4, Livonia, MI 48154-3367

1. Ⓐ Ⓑ Ⓒ Ⓓ

2. Ⓐ Ⓑ Ⓒ Ⓓ

3. Ⓐ Ⓑ Ⓒ Ⓓ

4. Ⓐ Ⓑ Ⓒ Ⓓ

5. Ⓐ Ⓑ Ⓒ Ⓓ

6. Ⓐ Ⓑ Ⓒ Ⓓ

7. Ⓐ Ⓑ Ⓒ Ⓓ

OFFICE USE ONLY

DATE RECEIVED

/ /

8. Ⓐ Ⓑ Ⓒ Ⓓ

GRADE

9. Ⓐ Ⓑ Ⓒ Ⓓ

10. Ⓐ Ⓑ Ⓒ Ⓓ

IIHIS   **A N S W E R   S H E E T**

INTERNATIONAL INSTITUTE FOR HEARING INSTRUMENTS STUDIES

DISTANCE LEARNING for Professionals in HEARING HEALTH SCIENCES

HEARING INSTRUMENT COMPONENTS AND CHARACTERISTICS

LESSON 23

FIFTH EDITION

STUDENT NUMBER

◀ Enter your five digit student number found on the inside front cover of this manual into the box at left.

■ Completely fill in the circle that indicates the correct answer.

■ Upon completion, tear out the answer sheet and return it for scoring to: IIHIS, 16880 Middlebelt Road, Suite 4, Livonia, MI 48154-3367

1. (A) (B) (C) (D)

2. (A) (B) (C) (D)

3. (A) (B) (C) (D)

4. (A) (B) (C) (D)

5. (A) (B) (C) (D)

6. (A) (B) (C) (D)

7. (A) (B) (C) (D)

8. (A) (B) (C) (D)

9. (A) (B) (C) (D)

10. (A) (B) (C) (D)

OFFICE USE ONLY

DATE RECEIVED

/ /

GRADE

IIHIS

ANSWER SHEET

INTERNATIONAL INSTITUTE FOR HEARING INSTRUMENTS STUDIES

DISTANCE LEARNING for Professionals in HEARING HEALTH SCIENCES

ANSI STANDARDS

LESSON 24

FIFTH EDITION

STUDENT NUMBER

◀ Enter your five digit student number found on the inside front cover of this manual into the box at left.

■ Completely fill in the circle that indicates the correct answer.

■ Upon completion, tear out the answer sheet and return it for scoring to: IIHIS, 16880 Middlebelt Road, Suite 4, Livonia, MI 48154-3367

1. Ⓐ Ⓑ Ⓒ Ⓓ

2. Ⓐ Ⓑ Ⓒ Ⓓ

3. Ⓐ Ⓑ Ⓒ Ⓓ

4. Ⓐ Ⓑ Ⓒ Ⓓ

5. Ⓐ Ⓑ Ⓒ Ⓓ

6. Ⓐ Ⓑ Ⓒ Ⓓ

7. Ⓐ Ⓑ Ⓒ Ⓓ

OFFICE USE ONLY

DATE RECEIVED

/ /

8. Ⓐ Ⓑ Ⓒ Ⓓ

GRADE

9. Ⓐ Ⓑ Ⓒ Ⓓ

10. Ⓐ Ⓑ Ⓒ Ⓓ

IIHIS   **ANSWER SHEET**

INTERNATIONAL INSTITUTE FOR HEARING INSTRUMENTS STUDIES

DISTANCE LEARNING for Professionals in HEARING HEALTH SCIENCES

EARMOLDS

LESSON 25

FIFTH EDITION

STUDENT NUMBER

◀ Enter your five digit student number found on the inside front cover of this manual into the box at left.

■ Completely fill in the circle that indicates the correct answer.

■ Upon completion, tear out the answer sheet and return it for scoring to: IIHIS, 16880 Middlebelt Road, Suite 4, Livonia, MI 48154-3367

1. Ⓐ Ⓑ Ⓒ Ⓓ

2. Ⓐ Ⓑ Ⓒ Ⓓ

3. Ⓐ Ⓑ Ⓒ Ⓓ

4. Ⓐ Ⓑ Ⓒ Ⓓ

5. Ⓐ Ⓑ Ⓒ Ⓓ

6. Ⓐ Ⓑ Ⓒ Ⓓ

7. Ⓐ Ⓑ Ⓒ Ⓓ

OFFICE USE ONLY

DATE RECEIVED

/   /

8. Ⓐ Ⓑ Ⓒ Ⓓ

GRADE

9. Ⓐ Ⓑ Ⓒ Ⓓ

10. Ⓐ Ⓑ Ⓒ Ⓓ

IIHIS **A N S W E R   S H E E T**

STUDENT NUMBER

◀ Enter your five digit student number found on the inside front cover of this manual into the box at left.

■ Completely fill in the circle that indicates the correct answer.

■ Upon completion, tear out the answer sheet and return it for scoring to: IIHIS, 16880 Middlebelt Road, Suite 4, Livonia, MI 48154-3367

1. Ⓐ   Ⓑ   Ⓒ   Ⓓ

2. Ⓐ   Ⓑ   Ⓒ   Ⓓ

3. Ⓐ   Ⓑ   Ⓒ   Ⓓ

4. Ⓐ   Ⓑ   Ⓒ   Ⓓ

5. Ⓐ   Ⓑ   Ⓒ   Ⓓ

6. Ⓐ   Ⓑ   Ⓒ   Ⓓ

7. Ⓐ   Ⓑ   Ⓒ   Ⓓ

8. Ⓐ   Ⓑ   Ⓒ   Ⓓ

9. Ⓐ   Ⓑ   Ⓒ   Ⓓ

10. Ⓐ   Ⓑ   Ⓒ   Ⓓ

OFFICE USE ONLY

DATE RECEIVED

/ /

GRADE

INTERNATIONAL INSTITUTE FOR HEARING INSTRUMENTS STUDIES

DISTANCE LEARNING for Professionals in HEARING HEALTH SCIENCES

FITTING VERIFICATION

LESSON 27

FIFTH EDITION

STUDENT NUMBER

◄ Enter your five digit student number found on the inside front cover of this manual into the box at left.

■ Completely fill in the circle that indicates the correct answer.

■ Upon completion, tear out the answer sheet and return it for scoring to: IIHIS, 16880 Middlebelt Road, Suite 4, Livonia, MI 48154-3367

1. Ⓐ Ⓑ Ⓒ Ⓓ

2. Ⓐ Ⓑ Ⓒ Ⓓ

3. Ⓐ Ⓑ Ⓒ Ⓓ

4. Ⓐ Ⓑ Ⓒ Ⓓ

5. Ⓐ Ⓑ Ⓒ Ⓓ

6. Ⓐ Ⓑ Ⓒ Ⓓ

7. Ⓐ Ⓑ Ⓒ Ⓓ

8. Ⓐ Ⓑ Ⓒ Ⓓ

9. Ⓐ Ⓑ Ⓒ Ⓓ

10. Ⓐ Ⓑ Ⓒ Ⓓ

INTERNATIONAL INSTITUTE FOR HEARING INSTRUMENTS STUDIES

DISTANCE LEARNING
for Professionals in
HEARING HEALTH SCIENCES

REAL EAR MEASUREMENT

LESSON 28

FIFTH EDITION

STUDENT NUMBER

◄ Enter your five digit student number found on the inside front cover of this manual into the box at left.

■ Completely fill in the circle that indicates the correct answer.

■ Upon completion, tear out the answer sheet and return it for scoring to: IIHIS, 16880 Middlebelt Road, Suite 4, Livonia, MI 48154-3367

1. Ⓐ Ⓑ Ⓒ Ⓓ

2. Ⓐ Ⓑ Ⓒ Ⓓ

3. Ⓐ Ⓑ Ⓒ Ⓓ

4. Ⓐ Ⓑ Ⓒ Ⓓ

5. Ⓐ Ⓑ Ⓒ Ⓓ

6. Ⓐ Ⓑ Ⓒ Ⓓ

7. Ⓐ Ⓑ Ⓒ Ⓓ

OFFICE USE ONLY

DATE RECEIVED

/   /

8. Ⓐ Ⓑ Ⓒ Ⓓ

GRADE

9. Ⓐ Ⓑ Ⓒ Ⓓ

10. Ⓐ Ⓑ Ⓒ Ⓓ

INTERNATIONAL INSTITUTE FOR HEARING INSTRUMENTS STUDIES

DISTANCE LEARNING for Professionals in HEARING HEALTH SCIENCES

POST FITTING CARE; FOLLOW-UP AND REHABILITATION

LESSON 29

FIFTH EDITION

STUDENT NUMBER

◀ Enter your five digit student number found on the inside front cover of this manual into the box at left.

■ Completely fill in the circle that indicates the correct answer.

■ Upon completion, tear out the answer sheet and return it for scoring to: IIHIS, 16880 Middlebelt Road, Suite 4, Livonia, MI 48154-3367

1. Ⓐ Ⓑ Ⓒ Ⓓ

2. Ⓐ Ⓑ Ⓒ Ⓓ

3. Ⓐ Ⓑ Ⓒ Ⓓ

4. Ⓐ Ⓑ Ⓒ Ⓓ

5. Ⓐ Ⓑ Ⓒ Ⓓ

6. Ⓐ Ⓑ Ⓒ Ⓓ

7. Ⓐ Ⓑ Ⓒ Ⓓ

OFFICE USE ONLY

DATE RECEIVED

/ /

8. Ⓐ Ⓑ Ⓒ Ⓓ

GRADE

9. Ⓐ Ⓑ Ⓒ Ⓓ

10. Ⓐ Ⓑ Ⓒ Ⓓ

IIHIS   **A N S W E R   S H E E T**